EASY KETOGENIC DIET SLOW COOKING

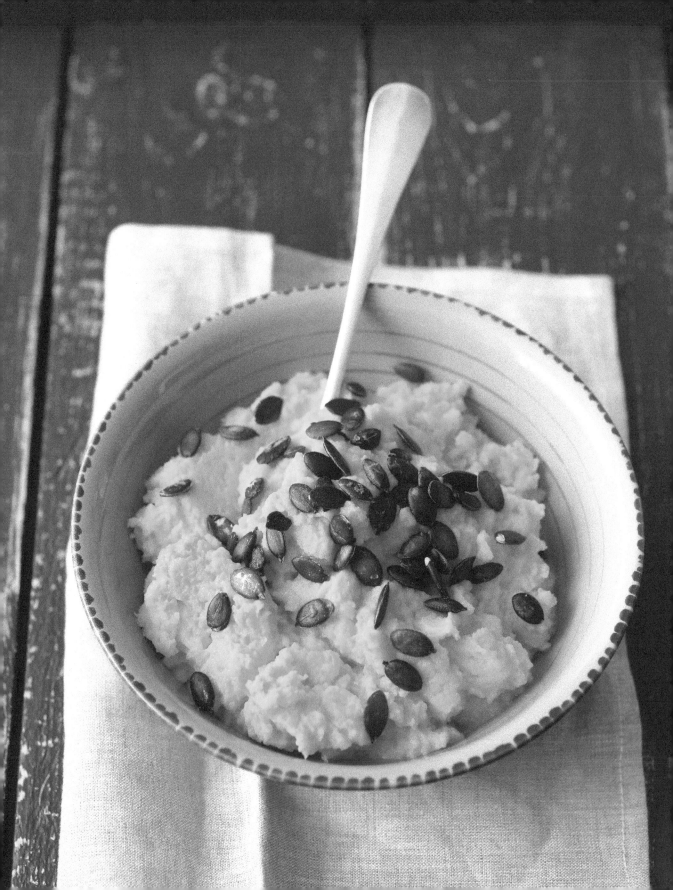

EASY
KETOGENIC DIET
SLOW COOKING

LOW-CARB, HIGH-FAT KETO RECIPES
THAT COOK THEMSELVES

AMY RAMOS

foreword by AMANDA C. HUGHES

ROCKRIDGE
PRESS

Photography © Nat & Cody Gantz, cover, pp. 42 & 116; Rua Castilho/Stockfood, p. ii; Meike Bergmann/Stockfood, p. viii; Jeff Wasserman/Stocksy, p. 12; Mikkel Adsbol/Stockfood, p. 22; Dan Jones/Stockfood, p. 62; PhotoCuisine/Thys/Supperdelux/StockFood, p. 80; Ashley Mackevicius/Stockfood, p. 98; Sporrer/Skowronek/Stockfood, p. 134; Gallo Images Pty Ltd./Stockfood, p. 152; Sandra Eckhardt/Stockfood, p. 170.

Cover Image: Simple Texas Chili, page 61
Title page image: Carrot-Pumpkin Pudding, page 65

ISBN: Print 978-1-62315-922-1 | eBook 978-1-62315-923-8

CONTENTS

FOREWORD

There are few things that excite me more than the words "slow cooker" before a recipe. Why? Because it brings to mind the idea of me walking into the house after a long day, climbing into my "house clothes" (see: not-real pants), opening the lid, and yelling, "Dinner's ready!"

Or, an exciting Sunday with my whole family sitting around the table, while I get to enjoy their company instead of sweating off my makeup and hairspray in the other room over a hot skillet.

On the ketogenic diet, one of the most common reasons why folks fall off the wagon is because they think it all requires blood, sweat, and keto tears. But really, it only requires a basic sense of the kitchen. For example, do you know how to turn the slow cooker on and off? You're doing great! Bravo! You don't have to be Thomas Keller or know how to juggle a zoodler and a jar of ghee with one hand. (Also, not recommended.)

Instead of going out to eat and spending $25–$100 on a so-called keto-friendly steak that's probably bathing in a seasoning of sugar and salt (this is actually a thing), I'm excited that the cookbook you're about to read is out in the wild for you to digest—not quite literally, but almost.

Because let's be honest—yes, keto takes some cooking. And it's entirely natural to get lazy and just want someone to spoon-feed you every once in a while. And you probably even could, with some of these recipes that are so simple even a toddler could cook them (although they're kind of boogery, so maybe you should just handle it).

That's the extra-nice thing about slow cooker meals. By the time you get home, you've totally forgotten about that prep you did earlier in the day. So you walk in all tired-eyed and less than bushy-tailed, but immediately smell something delicious. When you open the lid, it's like someone cooked you dinner—and it was you!

And that doesn't include the other sideline benefits, like making larger batches for lunches and leftovers, the ability to cook for a crowd, or making some dishes that taste scrumptious without turning your kitchen into a tornado. Can I get a high-five for fewer dishes?

What I love about this ketogenic slow cooker cookbook is that it will turn you into a little mini-expert on slow cooking. For example, did you know that you shouldn't cook seafood in the crockpot, or that herbs and dairy should always be added at the end? Did you know that frozen meats are a no-no? And do you know how to convert any normal recipe into a slow cooker recipe?

These were all topics I enjoyed learning about in this cookbook. You can even add a loaf pan to your slow cooker and make some pretty tasty breakfast loafs, like the Zucchini-Carrot Bread on page 24.

Another benefit of ketogenic slow cooking is soups, and this cookbook has no end to the number of soups you can make—from the Cheeseburger Soup on page 53 to the Chipotle Chicken Chili on page 60.

And a high-five to my veggie friends too, because there's a whole chapter for you. You'll find everything from a scrumptious Carrot-Pumpkin Pudding on page 65 to a Ratatouille on page 74. I love the use of pumpkin throughout the book, and especially in these recipes.

I hope you enjoy this cookbook as much as I did and that it keeps you feeling satisfied and energized on your ketogenic path—but at a slower, more relaxed pace.

Amanda C. Hughes
Keto Cook at WickedStuffed.com
Author of *Keto Life* and *The Wicked Good Ketogenic Diet Cookbook*

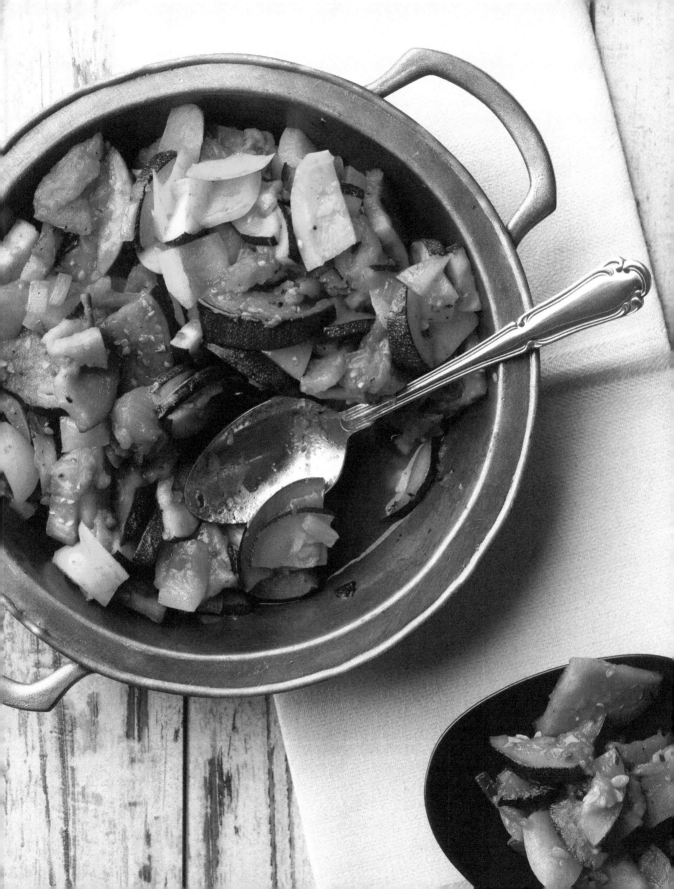

Chapter One
SLOW COOKING 101

Slow cookers are not new appliances in the culinary world. They have been around for decades; you might even have fond memories from your childhood of your parents serving your favorite dinner out of one. Slow cookers are very versatile because the cooking environment works the same no matter the cuisine. Knowing what slow cookers can and can't do is important for planning your meals, especially for a diet like keto.

In this chapter, you will learn slow-cooker basics such as which kind is best for your needs, how to ensure your recipes turn out great, and how to convert your traditional family favorites to work for you. Taking the mystery out of the slow cooker should give you the confidence to create spectacular keto meals as often as you want in order to reach your goals while eating well.

RATATOUILLE, PAGE 74

WHY SLOW COOK?

You might be wondering why you should invest in a slow cooker when other cooking techniques produce perfectly fine meals. Some of the reasons to use a slow cooker include:

- **Enhances flavor:** Cooking ingredients over several hours with spices, herbs, and other seasonings creates vegetables and proteins that burst with delicious flavors. This slow process allows the flavors to mellow and deepen for an enhanced eating experience.

- **Saves time:** Cooking at home takes a great deal of time: prepping, sautéing, stirring, turning the heat up and down, and watching the meal so that it does not over- or undercook. If you're unable to invest the time, you might find yourself reaching for convenience foods instead of healthy choices. Slow cookers allow you to do other activities while the meal cooks. You can put your ingredients in the slow cooker in the morning and come home to a perfectly cooked meal.

- **Convenient:** Besides the time-saving aspect, using a slow cooker can free up the stove and oven for other dishes. This can be very convenient for large holiday meals or when you want to serve a side dish and entrée as well as a delectable dessert. Clean up is simple when you use the slow cooker for messy meals because most inserts are nonstick or are easily cleaned with a little soapy water, and each meal is prepared in either just the machine or using one additional vessel to sauté ingredients. There is no wide assortment of pots, pans, and baking dishes to contend with at the end of the day.

- **Low heat production:** If you have ever cooked dinner on a scorching summer afternoon, you will appreciate the low amount of heat produced by a slow cooker. Even after eight hours of operation, slow cookers do not heat up your kitchen and you will not be sweating over the hot stovetop. Slow cookers use about a third of the energy of conventional cooking methods, just a little more energy than a traditional light bulb.

- **Supports healthy eating:** Cooking your food at high heat can reduce the nutrition profile of your foods, breaking down and removing the majority of vitamins, minerals, and antioxidants while producing unhealthy chemical compounds that can contribute to disease. Low-heat cooking retains all the goodness that you want for your diet.

- **Saves Money:** Slow cookers save you money because of the low amount of electricity they use and because the best ingredients for slow cooking are the less expensive cuts of beef and heartier inexpensive vegetables. Tougher cuts of meat—brisket, chuck, shanks—break down beautifully to fork-tender goodness. Another cost-saving benefit is that most 6-quart slow cookers will produce enough of a recipe to stretch your meals over at least two days. Leftovers are one of the best methods for saving money.

COOKING WITH HEAT AND STEAM

There are two methods for cooking food: moist or dry heat. Ovens, grills, and pan-frying use dry heat. Moist-heat methods include braising, stewing, and steaming. Slow cookers fall in the moist-heat category because of their low-temperature, closed-cooking environment. This method is perfect for tough cuts of meat and breaking down fibrous vegetables. Temperature and steam both come into play to create this favorable environment.

Temperature

Slow cookers feature a range of temperatures for convenience. Basic slow cookers have low and high settings, and more advanced models include digital displays for exact temperatures and probes that can be inserted. The recipes in this book are geared toward low-heat cooking, about 180°F to 200°F, so that any liquid simmers gently at a food-safe 185°F and the timing is long. The best temperature to create tender meats is 180°F; it is high enough for connective tissues to break down into tenderizing gelatin but low enough that the meat will not overcook. Low settings also allow you to assemble your recipe and then leave the house for a regular work-day while it cooks without compromising food quality or health.

High settings cook recipes approximately twice as fast. As a result, high-heat recipes can require some supervision to avoid overcooking meats or more delicate ingredients. Also, if you cook your food too fast, it might sit longer before you eat it, which is not safe. Two hours is the maximum time any recipe should be held on the "warm" setting. If you are planning to be home or need your meal quicker, then high heat in a slow cooker works fine for most recipes besides desserts and those that require baking.

Steam

Slow cookers have a tight-fitting lid that traps the steam created as the food cooks and the temperature heats up in the insert. The liquid in the slow cooker simmers creating steam, which very gently cooks the ingredients without compromising flavor and texture. As this steam is produced, this locked environment inhibits bacteria growth, so lifting the lid during the cooking process can be done once or twice to check progress, but multiple times is not recommended.

The steamy environment is limiting because it does not allow meats to brown, vegetables to caramelize, and the skin of poultry to crisp up. All of these effects require dry heat. So there are some recipes that aren't best for your slow cooker. For further reference, you can look at "When to Pass on the Crock" on page 6.

SLOW COOKER MYTHS

Slow cookers have been around for a long time, and most people have tried them at one point or another, sometimes successfully and other times not. When the results aren't perfect, false assumptions crop up. Some of the most common myths surrounding slow cookers are:

- **You can't open the lid.** This is a recommendation, but you can open the lid without ruining your meal. Lifting the lid will drop the temperature 15 to 30°F depending on how long the lid is off the insert. If done early in the timing, 2 to 3 hours in a 6-hour recipe, then you should extend the time 30 minutes. If you lift the lid near the end, it won't affect anything at all.

- **All the recipes taste the same.** Any type of cuisine, from South American to Indian, can be made in a slow cooker. Spices and flavors deepen in the slow cooker, so your meals should be more flavorful than standard cooking methods no matter what kind of food you are cooking. If your recipes all taste the same, you might be using similar recipes or seasonings.

- **You have to completely fill the insert.** Many slow cooker recipes produce a vast amount of food because the insert is filled completely. You don't have to do this. Filling the insert halfway or one-third of the way simply means adjusting the time to fewer hours. The more food in the insert, the more time on the timer.

- **You have to precook ingredients.** Precooking can be beneficial for certain types of ingredients, such as red meats and poultry with skin. However, you do not have to precook any of your ingredients at all. Browned meat and chicken are more attractive and have a richer flavor than meat that hasn't been browned, but there isn't a vast difference between the two. You will still enjoy a delicious meal if you skip this step. It's a good idea to remove poultry skin though, because the texture is a little unpleasant without time in the skillet.

- **You're limited to stews and casseroles.** Slow cookers are incredibly versatile, and recipes have come a long way over the decades. Desserts, breads, side dishes, glazed meats, and even granola can be made effectively in a slow cooker with fabulous results. Soups, stews, chili, and braised meats are still slow-cooker staples because they turn out particularly well, but you can make almost anything—and make it delicious.

Slow cookers are wonderful for many types of dishes, but they certainly cannot be used for everything you will eat on the keto diet. Obviously, grilled and broiled meats are impossible because delicious caramelization is not possible with a slow cooker. This is why precooking is recommended for some meats and poultry. You can bake in the slow cooker, but the browning that occurs in dry heat will not happen. As stated elsewhere in this book, recipes that incorporate dairy products from the beginning of a recipe do not turn out well. The long cooking times in slow cookers causes dairy to split, and you end up with lumps of whey bound to casein. Here are some foods and dishes that are not ideally suited for slow cookers:

- Tender cuts of meat such as beef sirloin or beef tenderloin

- Seafood

- Delicate vegetables such as asparagus or lettuces (unless added at the very end)

- Fresh herbs (unless added at the very end)

- Dairy products (unless added at the very end)

THE RIGHT COOKER FOR YOU

Slow cookers have changed a lot over the years. These days you can purchase models that range from very simple models all the way to ones that look like they should be on a space station. When buying the right model for your needs, you have to consider what you are cooking, how many portions, and if you will be home during the cooking process. All these factors are important when deciding on the size, shape, and features of your slow cooker.

Size and Shape

Slow cookers come in a multitude of sizes and shapes, so it is important to con-sider your needs and what will work best for the type of food prepared on the keto diet. There are models that range from ½-quart to large 8-quart models and everything in-between.

The small slow cookers (½-quart to 2-quart) are usually used for dips or sauces, as well as recipes designed for one person. Medium-sized slow cookers (3-quart to 4-quart) are great for baking or for meals that create food for two to three people. The slow cooker recommended for most of the recipes in this book is the 5-quart to 6-quart model because it is perfect for the large cuts of meat on the keto diet and can prepare food for four people, including leftovers. The enormous 7-quart to 8-quart appliance is meant for very large meals. If you have money in your budget, owning both a 3-quart and 6-quart model would be the best of both worlds.

When it comes to shapes, you will have to decide between round, oval, and rectangular. Round slow cookers are fine for stews and chili, but do not work well for large pieces of meat. These should probably not be your choice. Oval and rectangular slow cookers both allow for the ingredients you will use regularly that are large, like roasts, ribs, and chops, and have the added advantage of fitting loaf pans, ramekins, and casserole dishes, as well. Some desserts and breads are best cooked in another container placed in the slow cooker, and you will see several recipes in this book that use that technique.

Features

Now that you know the size and shape of the recommended slow cooker, it is time to consider what you want this appliance to do for you. Depending on your budget, at a minimum you want a slow cooker with temperature controls that cover warm, low, and high, as well as a removable insert. These are the primary features of the bare-bones models that will get the job done. However, if you want to truly experience a set-it-and-forget-it appliance that creates the best meals possible in this cooking environment, you might want to consider the following features:

- **Digital programmable controls:** You can program temperature, when the slow cooker starts, how long it cooks, and when the slow cooker switches to warm.

- **Glass lid:** These are heavier, and allow you to look into the slow cooker without removing them, so there is little heat loss. Opt for a lid with clamps, and you can transport your cooked meal easily to parties and gatherings if needed.

If you opt for a basic, analog slow cooker—the kind with a dial—or already have one that is not programmable, there is still an option if you want to control the cooking time. This might be something to consider if you are usually away from your home more than the time needed for the recipes you are cooking. A socket timer—the same kind that people use to switch their lights on and off when on vacation—is a great hack to turn your basic slow cooker into a programmable model. You simply plug your slow cooker into it, turn your slow cooker to the desired high or low setting, and set the timer for how long the cooking process should take, and when you want it to turn on or off. This timer will only work if you have a slow cooker that is set with a dial because a digital model needs to be manually set when turned on. For food-safety reasons, the ingredients need to be completely chilled in the insert until you are ready to leave the house and the timer should not be set for prolonged periods of time.

- **Temperature probe:** Once you have a slow cooker with this feature, you will wonder how you cooked previously without it. The temperature probe allows you to cook your meat, poultry, and egg dishes to an exact temperature and then switches to warm when completed.

- **Precooking feature:** Some models have a precooking feature that allows you to brown your meat and poultry right in the insert. You will still have to take the time to do this step, but you won't have a skillet to clean afterward.

10 TIPS FOR SLOW-COOKING SUCCESS

Slow cookers are simple to use, but you can increase your success with a few tips and techniques. In the following list, some tips are suggestions and some should be considered more seriously for safety or health reasons. The intent is to provide the best information possible so that your meals are delicious and easy.

Always

1. **Read the user manual and any other literature.** You will find an assortment of instructions included in the slow-cooker box so take the time to sit down and read everything completely before using a new device. You might think you know how everything works, but each model is a little different and it is best to be informed about all of the things your slow cooker can do.

2. **Grease the insert of the slow cooker before cooking.** Cleaning a slow cooker insert can be a challenge, so grease the insert, even for soups and stews. You don't want to scrub the insert with abrasive brushes or scraping bits of cooked-on food off, because you will wreck its nonstick surface.

3. **Add dairy and herbs at the end of the cooking process.** As stated elsewhere in this book, dairy and fresh herbs do not hold up well during long cooking times. Dairy splits and creates a grainy, unpleasant texture, and herbs lose their flavor, color, and texture. Always add these ingredients at the end.

4. **Always cut your ingredients into similar-sized pieces.** Slow cookers are not meant to be used for staggered cooking recipes such as stir-fries where the more delicate ingredients are added last to avoid overcooking. Evenly sized pieces mean your ingredients will be ready at the same time and your meals will be cooked evenly.

5. **Adjust your seasonings.** Slow cookers can have an unexpected effect on herbs and spices so it is important to taste and adjust at the end of the process. Some spices, such as curry or cayenne, can get more intense, while the long cooking time can reduce the impact of dried herbs. It is best to hold off on too much salt until the very end as well because it will get stronger.

Never

1. **Add too much liquid.** Very little evaporation occurs in a slow cooker compared to stovetop or oven cooking. Most slow cooker recipes, with the exception of soups and sauces, call for 50 percent less liquid than conventional ones.

2. **Use frozen meats or poultry.** The ingredients in slow cookers need to reach 140°F within 4 hours for food safety, so large cuts of meat or poultry should be fully thawed. You can add small frozen items like meatballs to a slow cooker because these can come to temperature within this time range.

3. **Place your insert right from the refrigerator into the slow cooker.** When you remove your previously prepared meal from the refrigerator, let the insert sit out at room temperature for 30 minutes or so to avoid cracking it with extreme temperature changes. Also, never remove the hot insert from your slow cooker and place it on a cold surface.

4. **Resume cooking after a power outage of over two hours.** Power outages can happen in any season, and for food-safety reasons, you have to err on the side of caution. If an outage lasts for more than two hours, especially during the first few hours of the cooking time, you need to discard the food because the amount of time spent in the food danger zone (40°F to 140°F) will have been too long. If the outage is less than two hours and it occurs after your food has been cooking for at least four hours, then you can resume cooking until the end of the original time or transfer the food to a pot or casserole dish and finish it on the stove or in the oven. When in doubt, throw the food out.

5. **Use the recommended cooking times in high altitudes.** As with most other cooking methods, slow cookers need more cooking time if you live above an altitude of 3,000 feet. The liquid in the slow cooker will simmer at a lower temperature so high-heat settings are recommended, or if you can program the slow cooker, then set it to maintain the food at 200°F or higher. You can also use a temperature probe set to 165°F internal temperature if your slow cooker has this feature.

CONVERTING A FAVORITE RECIPE TO THE SLOW COOKER

If you have a recipe that is a tried-and-true family favorite, you might be able to convert it for your slow cooker. Obviously, if you are trying to adapt Uncle Bob's famous grilled beef tenderloin, you might be out of luck. Take a look at the type of recipe and follow a few simple guidelines to convert it to a convenient slow-cooker version. These guidelines include:

- Don't try recipes that require less than 15 minutes of cooking time because the ingredients will probably not hold up well enough.

- Reduce the amount of liquid in the recipe, unless you are making a soup, because the sealed environment of a slow cooker creates a steaming effect where the liquid condenses on the lid and falls back into the insert. Use about half of the recommended liquid.

- If the recipe does not ask for any liquid, as is the case with roasted joints of meat or poultry, add between ¼ cup and ½ cup of water or broth.

- Leave out any dairy products until the end of the cooking time, or if the product is used as the only liquid, then replace it with coconut milk.

- Brown your meats and poultry so that you get the same rich flavor and gorgeous color.

- Make sure to convert the recipe's cook time to work with a slow cooker: 15 minutes equals 1 to 2 hours on low, 30 minutes equals 3 to 4 hours on low, 45 minutes equals 5 to 6 hours on low, 1 hour equals 6 to 8 hours on low, and 2 hours equals 9 to 10 hours on low.

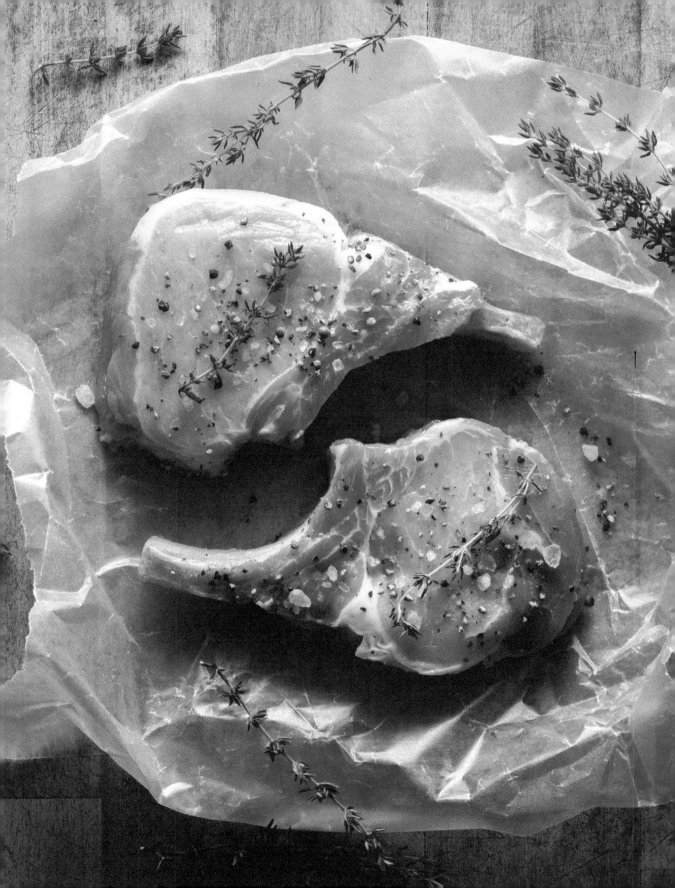

Chapter Two

COOK FOOD SLOW, BURN FAT FAST

Now that you know all about slow cookers and how to use them effectively, you can delve into why this handy appliance is a stellar choice for the keto diet. Keto definitely requires meal planning and selecting your ingredients carefully for the most positive impact on your health and weight. Slow cookers can help you plan more efficiently, and the cooking method suits the keto parameters beautifully. You can create delectable keto meals easily for immediate enjoyment or create containers of leftovers to consume later in the week. You will wonder how you ever followed the keto diet so well without a slow cooker after trying it for a couple weeks.

KETO AND THE COOKER

Following a diet to lose weight can be incredibly difficult at first. Keto is no different; it is a strict eating plan with very little wiggle room. The first few months of the keto diet can be exciting because of initial weight-loss success since eliminating refined sugar and processed foods can seriously impact your weight. Sticking to the plan can be difficult due to time constraints and commitments in your life. A slow cooker allows you to create keto-compliant meals without too much effort. Slow cookers work well with the ingredients in the keto diet such as:

- **Healthy fats:** The type of food that slow cookers produce incorporates many of the healthy fats that are so important to the keto plan. Soups, stews, roasts, chili, and luscious desserts can be enhanced by and topped with ingredients such as coconut milk, heavy (whipping) cream, full-fat cheeses, yogurt, and avocado. You will have no problem staying in your keto macros with a slow cooker.

- **Lots of protein:** Keto is very meat and poultry heavy because moderate protein, between 20 and 25 percent of calories, requires including some sort of meat or poultry in every meal. Slow cookers excel at roasts, ribs, chicken, and meatloaf. You can also create delicious egg dishes for breakfast that can cook all night for convenience.

- **Whole foods:** The core of the keto diet is home-prepared meals that feature whole foods rather than convenience foods. Cooking every meal from scratch is a massive undertaking and requires precision meal planning to successfully pull off long term. Slow cookers allow you to use whole, nutritious foods like meats, vegetables that grow above the ground, eggs, and healthy fats easily in delicious combinations.

Fat bombs are snacks or treats that are extremely high in fat and low in carbs. They cannot be made in a slow cooker, but you can use these luscious morsels to balance your keto macros. Fat bombs can be savory or sweet, depending on your preference, and are composed of healthy fats such as grass-fed butter, coconut oil, or nut butters. They are flavored with extracts or cocoa powder and often contain texture-adding ingredients such as unsweetened shredded coconut, nuts, or seeds.

MEAL PLANNING AND MAKING AHEAD

Cooking healthy meals for a family or just for yourself every week can be a daunting task, even when you are not trying to follow a specific diet plan like keto. Planning your meals can sometimes make the difference between a successful week and food choices that are not ideal. The trick to good meal planning is knowing what your week looks like with respect to time and combining ingredients over multiple meals to save money. A slow cooker effortlessly produces some of your meals and allows you to create leftovers for other meals on days when you do not have time to cook. Below are some helpful meal-planning tips to help you stick to your food and weight goals:

- **Use ingredients in more than one recipe.** Professional chefs use this trick to save money and time when designing a new menu. Ingredients such as ground beef or chopped onions that span several recipes can be purchased for less in large amounts. This will save time shopping and preparing the recipes. Make sure you divide items such as large packages of beef into the portions required for each recipe.

- **Batch cook on the weekend or your day off.** You can prepare an entire week's worth of food in one day with a little planning and a slow cooker. Then you freeze the meals for later in the week and store the other meals in the refrigerator in sealed containers for the first couple of days. You can cook one recipe overnight and create at least two others during the day in 6-hour cycles with a little cleanup in-between each meal.

- **Buy commonly used ingredients in bulk and when they are on sale.** You should certainly always have a shopping list but never pass up a fabulous deal on items you use all the time such as chicken breasts or chuck roasts. Also, think about buying a whole fresh chicken or turkey and butchering it into different cuts yourself to save money. The extra parts can be frozen for up to 3 months.

- **Prep some of your ingredients in advance.** If you don't have the time to batch cook your meals, you can prepare some of your ingredients in advance; for instance, storing prechopped onions and vegetables, and precooking meat or poultry. This saves time on the day you make the recipe, and most ingredients lose very little of their quality when stored in sealed containers in the refrigerator for a couple of days.

THE KETO-SLOW COOKER KITCHEN

Most of the ingredients in the keto diet work beautifully in a slow cooker, so if you have already converted your kitchen and pantry to be keto friendly, you won't have to make too many changes. The meats that are best suited to this preparation are the less-expensive cuts that are well marbled with collagen, which converts to gelatin as the meat cooks. The following ingredients are a great place to start your slow-cooker experience:

Meat

- Beef brisket, point cut (2 to 4 pounds)
- Chicken drumsticks (skin on)
- Chicken thighs (skin on)
- Chuck roast (2 to 4 pounds)
- Ground beef (80% protein/20% fat)
- Ground chicken
- Ground turkey
- Lamb shanks (2 to 3 pounds)
- Pork baby back ribs (2 to 3 pounds)
- Pork shoulder (or butt) (3 to 4 pounds)
- Short ribs (2 to 3 pounds)
- Whole chicken (3 to 5 pounds)

Vegetables and Fruits

- Bell peppers
- Blackberries
- Blueberries
- Broccoli
- Cabbage
- Carrots (in moderation)
- Cauliflower
- Celery
- Coconut
- Garlic (in moderation)
- Green beans
- Lemons
- Limes
- Mushrooms
- Okra
- Olives

Full-fat dairy and grass-fed butter are allowed on the keto diet and are often instrumental in adding the desired fat, texture, and delectable flavor to recipes. Unfortunately, dairy does not do well in slow cookers, except butter, so you have to be careful about when you add these ingredients. If you throw a dairy product in with all the other ingredients at the beginning, it will curdle as the meal cooks. Cheeses and heavy cream can be stirred into your egg casseroles with very little effect, especially if the timing is shorter, such as 4 to 6 hours on low. Cheese and cream can also be used from the beginning of the process in the case of cheesecakes and custards. The best time to whisk in heavy cream, sour cream, cream cheese, yogurt, and cheeses is at the very end of the cooking time, just before serving.

- Onions (in moderation)
- Pumpkin
- Raspberries
- Spaghetti squash (in moderation)
- Strawberries
- Tomatoes (in moderation)
- Zucchini

Fats

- Almond milk (unsweetened)
- Avocado oil
- Coconut cream, oil, milk, and unsweetened shredded
- Extra-virgin olive oil
- Full-fat dairy cheese, cream cheese, Greek yogurt, heavy [whipping] cream, sour cream
- Ghee (clarified butter)
- Grass-fed butter
- Lard
- Nut butters (almond, hazelnut, macadamia, peanut) with no added sugar
- Nuts and seeds and their oils (almonds, Brazil nuts, flaxseed, hazelnuts, macadamias, peanuts, pecans, pumpkin seeds, sunflower seeds, walnuts)
- Sesame oil

Herbs and Spices

- Allspice
- Anise seed
- Basil
- Bay leaf
- Caraway seed
- Cardamom
- Celery seed
- Chili powder
- Cinnamon, ground
- Cloves, ground
- Cumin seed
- Curry powder

- Ginger, ground
- Marjoram, dried
- Mustard seed
- Nutmeg
- Oregano
- Paprika
- Rosemary
- Sage
- Tarragon
- Thyme
- Turmeric

Delicate fresh herbs such as basil, parsley, and tarragon should be added at the end of the cooking time because they lose flavor and color when exposed to heat for hours and hours. Dried herbs and spices can intensify when used in a slow cooker, so if your palate prefers blander foods, start with half the amount of the seasonings and adjust them at the end.

ABOUT THE RECIPES

This book contains recipes that have many delicious ingredients that are allowed on the keto diet plan, including meats, protein, and seafood, as well as cruciferous vegetables, dark leafy greens, full-fat dairy, nuts, seeds, and berries. The best options are whole foods at the best quality you can find that suit your budget. They are all low-carb choices, so there are no recipes in this book with more than 10g net carbs, and more than 80 percent of the recipes, have 5g or less net carbs. The general guideline for keto is to stay under about 20g carbs per day. You will see

One of the biggest criticisms of slow cookers is that some of the ingredients need to be precooked for better results. This is why some slow cookers allow you to precook right in the insert to keep dirty skillets and pots to a minimum. If you own a slow cooker with no precooking setting, you can certainly just dump all the ingredients into the insert, turn the slow cooker on and walk away, and still have quite a nice meal at the end of the day. However, precooking some ingredients is recommended, especially meats and poultry. As stated earlier, slow cookers do not brown meat or crisp the skin on poultry. Searing meat creates the lovely coloring and rich flavor that is a desired component of the dish.

Poultry with skin needs to be seared also, or you will end up with flabby, pale skin pieces in your meal. Browned chicken skin is probably one of the tastiest parts of the whole bird, and this is reflected in the flavor of the finished recipe. Some vegetables, such as onions and garlic, can benefit from a little time in a skillet as well. This step can be done very quickly while you brown your meats and poultry. If you do not think you will have time in the morning to precook anything, just prepare the recipe the night before and leave the insert in the refrigerator. Let the insert sit out at room temperature for at least 30 minutes until you are ready to leave the house, and pop it in the slow cooker.

natural sweeteners in the recipes such as stevia and erythritol. Stevia is extracted from the leaves of a South American plant, and it is about 100 times sweeter than refined sugar and has no calories. Erythritol is a sugar alcohol that is low calorie and does not cause spikes in blood sugar. One of the most popular brands of erythritol is Swerve, which is found in most supermarkets and easily online.

The recipes do not contain most fruits, legumes, ingredients that contain gluten, pseudo grains, regular or low-fat dairy, or soy products. The coconut milk is full-fat and canned, and any processed ingredients, such as canned tomatoes or almond milk, are unsweetened and sodium-free.

You will notice that each recipe includes a keto quotient (high ◎, medium ◉, and low ●) and macros (fat/protein/carbs). Ideally, your calorie intake should be 70 percent or more from fat, 20 to 25 percent from protein, and 5 to 10 percent from carbs. A recipe with a high keto quotient has a higher fat percentage and protein and carbs in the acceptable range. A medium quotient means the recipe has a lower fat percentage but is still within the correct numbers, and its protein and carbs are in the desired range. A low keto quotient is when the fat percentage is below 70 percent, or the carbs are higher.

The recipes in the following chapters use ingredients that are packed with nutrients and selected specifically for the keto diet. Each recipe will be labeled with one or more of the following categories so you can pick the dishes that suit your needs.

- **Dairy-Free:** These recipes do not contain any milk products.

- **Nut-Free:** These recipes do not contain any nuts or nut products.

- **Allergen-Free:** These recipes do not contain any of the Big 8 allergens: milk, eggs, fish, crustacean shellfish, tree nuts, peanuts, wheat, or soybean.

- **Paleo-Friendly:** The ingredients in these recipes conform to the Paleo diet.

- **Quick Prep:** Preparation for these recipes takes 15 minutes or less.

The nutritional calculations for each recipe are just a guide; they can fluctuate depending on specific ingredient brands, the size of vegetables, and the cut or trim of your protein choices. It is important to consider your daily macros rather than get caught up in each calorie or carb gram. Food should still be delicious and fun to create.

RULES FOR FREEZING SLOW-COOKED FOOD

One of the benefits of a slow cooker is that with very little effort you can create large quantities of food that can be frozen for future meals. The best recipes to freeze are soups, stews, chili, meats with lots of sauce, meatloaf, and meatballs. Freezing food is not difficult, but there certainly are some ground rules to ensure food safety and the best quality when you thaw the meal out.

- Always chill the food completely in the refrigerator before placing the sealed container in the freezer so you don't get extensive condensation in the container that freezes into damaging ice crystals.

- Whenever possible, if there is a sauce in the meal, make sure it covers the protein or other ingredients to prevent freezer burn, and remove any air from the freezer bags, if using them.

- Some ingredients, such as tender vegetables like green beans or asparagus, do not freeze well, so it is best to leave them out of the recipe completely.

- Leave out certain dairy products if you plan to freeze a meal; wait until you thaw the meal at a future time and whisk in the appropriate amount of heavy cream, sour cream, or yogurt when the meal is reheated.

- Thaw your frozen recipes in the refrigerator, not at room temperature.

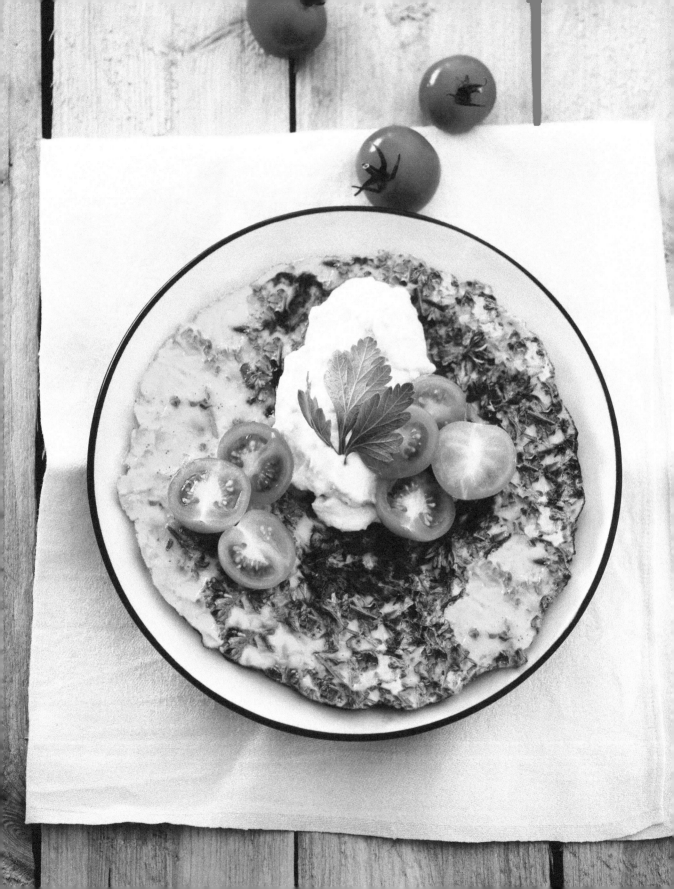

← SPANAKOPITA FRITTATA, PAGE 36

ZUCCHINI-CARROT BREAD

MAKES 8 SLICES / PREP TIME: 15 MINUTES / COOK TIME: 3 HOURS ON HIGH OR 5 HOURS ON LOW

DAIRY-FREE
QUICK PREP

KETO QUOTIENT

MACRONUTRIENTS
72% FAT
18% PROTEIN
10% CARBS

PER SERVING (1 SLICE)
CALORIES: 217
TOTAL FAT: 19G
PROTEIN: 8G
TOTAL CARBS: 5G
FIBER: 3G
NET CARBS: 2G
CHOLESTEROL: 136MG

Zucchini is a fantastic garden vegetable that seems to multiply overnight in my backyard garden. This recipe creates a moist, flavorful loaf that isn't as dense as bread. This version is warmly spiced and gets its moisture from carrots. Try a slice for breakfast with a generous smear of butter to complement its consistency.

2 TEASPOONS BUTTER, FOR GREASING PAN

1 CUP ALMOND FLOUR

1 CUP GRANULATED ERYTHRITOL

½ CUP COCONUT FLOUR

1½ TEASPOONS BAKING POWDER

1 TEASPOON GROUND CINNAMON

½ TEASPOON GROUND NUTMEG

½ TEASPOON BAKING SODA

¼ TEASPOON SALT

4 EGGS

½ CUP BUTTER, MELTED

1 TABLESPOON PURE VANILLA EXTRACT

1½ CUPS FINELY GRATED ZUCCHINI

½ CUP FINELY GRATED CARROT

1. Lightly grease a 9-by-5-inch loaf pan with the butter and set aside.

2. Place a small rack in the bottom of your slow cooker.

3. In a large bowl, stir together the almond flour, erythritol, coconut flour, baking powder, cinnamon, nutmeg, baking soda, and salt until well mixed.

4. In a separate medium bowl, whisk together the eggs, melted butter, and vanilla until well blended.

5. Add the wet ingredients to dry ingredients and stir to combine.

6. Stir in the zucchini and carrot.

7. Spoon the batter into the prepared loaf pan.

8. Place the loaf pan on the rack in the bottom of the slow cooker, cover, and cook on high for 3 hours.

9. Remove the loaf pan, let the bread cool completely, and serve.

ALLERGEN TIP: If you have an allergy to tree nuts, you can replace the almond flour with ¼ cup coconut flour, increasing the amount in the recipe to ¾ cup. This means increasing the eggs to 5 in total as well.

KETO GRANOLA

SERVES 16 / PREP TIME: 10 MINUTES / COOK TIME: 3 TO 4 HOURS ON LOW

Granola is incredibly versatile. It can be eaten as a breakfast cereal with a splash of almond milk, as a lovely topping for a creamy bowl of yogurt, or as a crunchy snack on its own. The hints of maple and cinnamon in this recipe elevate a delicious product to something that might become addictive if you aren't careful. The serving size is small, but keep in mind that a little will fill you up.

½ CUP COCONUT OIL, MELTED

2 TEASPOONS PURE VANILLA EXTRACT

1 TEASPOON MAPLE EXTRACT

1 CUP CHOPPED PECANS

1 CUP SUNFLOWER SEEDS

1 CUP UNSWEETENED SHREDDED COCONUT

½ CUP HAZELNUTS

½ CUP SLIVERED ALMONDS

¼ CUP GRANULATED ERYTHRITOL

½ TEASPOON CINNAMON

¼ TEASPOON GROUND NUTMEG

¼ TEASPOON SALT

1. Lightly grease the insert of the slow cooker with 1 tablespoon of the coconut oil.

2. In a large bowl, whisk together the remaining coconut oil, vanilla, and maple extract. Add the pecans, sunflower seeds, coconut, hazelnuts, almonds, erythritol, cinnamon, nutmeg, and salt. Toss to coat the nuts and seeds.

3. Transfer the mixture to the insert.

4. Cover and cook on low for 3 to 4 hours, until the granola is crispy.

5. Transfer the granola to a baking sheet covered in parchment or foil to cool.

6. Store in a sealed container in the refrigerator for up to 2 weeks.

> **VARIATION TIP:** Granola recipes are quite flexible because the combination of nuts, seeds, and spices will taste great no matter what the proportion. Substitute different nuts or spices to suit your palate as long as you use the same finishing amounts, about 4 cups in total.

DAIRY-FREE
QUICK PREP

KETO QUOTIENT

MACRONUTRIENTS
84% FAT
10% PROTEIN
6% CARBS

PER SERVING (⅓ CUP)
CALORIES: 236
TOTAL FAT: 23G
PROTEIN: 6G
TOTAL CARBS: 5G
FIBER: 3G
NET CARBS: 2G
CHOLESTEROL: 0MG

PUMPKIN-PIE BREAKFAST BARS

MAKES 8 BARS / PREP TIME: 15 MINUTES / COOK TIME: 3 HOURS ON LOW

QUICK PREP

KETO QUOTIENT

MACRONUTRIENTS
72% FAT
15% PROTEIN
13% CARBS

PER SERVING
CALORIES: 227
TOTAL FAT: 19G
PROTEIN: 10G
TOTAL CARBS: 8G
FIBER: 4G
NET CARBS: 4G
CHOLESTEROL: 143MG

Commercially prepared grab-and-go breakfast bars are filled with sugar and preservatives, but these easy-to-prepare beauties will start your day off right with whole-food ingredients and a satisfying hint of sweetness. You might even feel guilty because they taste like a decadent dessert rather than a healthy meal choice. Don't just save these bars for breakfast: They make a wonderful midmorning or afternoon snack as well.

FOR THE CRUST

5 TABLESPOONS BUTTER, SOFTENED, DIVIDED

¾ CUP UNSWEETENED SHREDDED COCONUT

½ CUP ALMOND FLOUR

¼ CUP GRANULATED ERYTHRITOL

FOR THE FILLING

1 (28-OUNCE) CAN PUMPKIN PURÉE

1 CUP HEAVY (WHIPPING) CREAM

4 EGGS

1 OUNCE PROTEIN POWDER

1 TEASPOON PURE VANILLA EXTRACT

4 DROPS LIQUID STEVIA

1 TEASPOON GROUND CINNAMON

½ TEASPOON GROUND GINGER

¼ TEASPOON GROUND NUTMEG

PINCH GROUND CLOVES

PINCH SALT

For the crust

1. Lightly grease the bottom of the insert of the slow cooker with 1 tablespoon of the butter.

2. In a small bowl, stir together the coconut, almond flour, erythritol, and remaining butter until the mixture forms into coarse crumbs.

3. Press the crumbs into the bottom of the insert evenly to form a crust.

For the filling

1. In a medium bowl, stir together the pumpkin, heavy cream, eggs, protein powder, vanilla, stevia, cinnamon, ginger, nutmeg, cloves, and salt until well blended.

2. Spread the filling evenly over the crust.

3. Cover and cook on low for 3 hours.

4. Uncover and let cool for 30 minutes. Then place the insert in the refrigerator until completely chilled, about 2 hours.

5. Cut into squares and store them in the refrigerator in a sealed container for up to 5 days.

> **ALLERGEN TIP:** Milk allergies include ingredients like butter and heavy cream, which are often used in delicious bars and baking. If you are allergic to dairy, replace the butter with coconut oil and the heavy cream with coconut milk.

NUTTY "OATMEAL"

SERVES 6 / PREP TIME: 10 MINUTES / COOK TIME: 8 HOURS ON LOW

You might wonder what an avocado is doing in this hot cereal recipe. It's because this nutrient-dense fruit adds a luscious richness and a creamy texture. The hefty amount of healthy fats and antioxidants in avocado also balances the keto-macronutrient ratio.

1 TABLESPOON COCONUT OIL

1 CUP COCONUT MILK

1 CUP UNSWEETENED SHREDDED COCONUT

½ CUP CHOPPED PECANS

½ CUP SLICED ALMONDS

¼ CUP GRANULATED ERYTHRITOL

1 AVOCADO, DICED

2 OUNCES PROTEIN POWDER

1 TEASPOON GROUND CINNAMON

¼ TEASPOON GROUND NUTMEG

½ CUP BLUEBERRIES, FOR GARNISH

1. Lightly grease the insert of a slower cooker with the coconut oil.

2. Place the coconut milk, shredded coconut, pecans, almonds, erythritol, avocado, protein powder, cinnamon, and nutmeg in the slow cooker.

3. Cover and cook on low for 8 hours.

4. Stir the mixture to create the desired texture.

5. Serve topped with the blueberries.

ALLERGEN TIP: If you have an egg sensitivity or soy allergy, you have to be very vigilant when selecting protein powder. Find a product that is made from hemp or rice sources, usually in the vegan or organic section of the supermarket.

PUMPKIN-PECAN N'OATMEAL

SERVES 4 / PREP TIME: 10 MINUTES / COOK TIME: 8 HOURS ON LOW

Many people enjoy starting their day with a steaming bowl of oatmeal and miss the comfort of this filling hot breakfast when they start following the keto diet. Ground nuts, sweet pumpkin, and a hint of maple flavor combine to create the perfect n'oatmeal. The best part is you can make this dish overnight if you are an early riser! Try different toppings such as chopped hazelnuts, your favorite berries, or a spoon of unsweetened shredded coconut to create fabulous variations.

DAIRY-FREE
QUICK PREP

KETO QUOTIENT

MACRONUTRIENTS
80% FAT
15% PROTEIN
5% CARBS

PER SERVING
CALORIES: 292
TOTAL FAT: 26G
PROTEIN: 10G
TOTAL CARBS: 9G
FIBER: 2G
NET CARBS: 7G
CHOLESTEROL: 0MG

1 TABLESPOON COCONUT OIL

3 CUPS CUBED PUMPKIN, CUT INTO
   1-INCH CHUNKS

2 CUPS COCONUT MILK

½ CUP GROUND PECANS

1 OUNCE PLAIN PROTEIN POWDER

2 TABLESPOONS GRANULATED ERYTHRITOL

1 TEASPOON MAPLE EXTRACT

½ TEASPOON GROUND NUTMEG

¼ TEASPOON GROUND CINNAMON

PINCH GROUND ALLSPICE

1. Lightly grease the insert of a slower cooker with the coconut oil.

2. Place the pumpkin, coconut milk, pecans, protein powder, erythritol, maple extract, nutmeg, cinnamon, and allspice in the insert.

3. Cover and cook on low for 8 hours.

4. Stir the mixture or use a potato masher to create your preferred texture, and serve.

ALLERGEN TIP: If you are allergic to nuts, simply replace the ground pecans with unsweetened shredded coconut and make sure you are using a plant-based protein powder, either hemp or rice based. This will slightly lessen the fat and increase the protein, but will still keep them within the keto range.

PUMPKIN-NUTMEG PUDDING

SERVES 8 / PREP TIME: 15 MINUTES / COOK TIME: 6 TO 7 HOURS ON LOW

In Europe, custards and hot creamy puddings are often served for breakfast. This version has a gorgeous golden color and tastes like a perfect pumpkin pie without the crust. It is lovely served warm or chilled, and can be topped with whipped cream, toasted pumpkin seeds, pecans, or fresh berries if you want to impress those who you are sharing it with.

¼ CUP MELTED BUTTER, DIVIDED

2½ CUPS CANNED PUMPKIN PURÉE

2 CUPS COCONUT MILK

4 EGGS

1 TABLESPOON PURE VANILLA EXTRACT

1 CUP ALMOND FLOUR

½ CUP GRANULATED ERYTHRITOL

2 OUNCES PROTEIN POWDER

1 TEASPOON BAKING POWDER

1 TEASPOON GROUND CINNAMON

¼ TEASPOON GROUND NUTMEG

PINCH GROUND CLOVES

1. Lightly grease the insert of the slow cooker with 1 tablespoon of the butter.

2. In a large bowl, whisk together the remaining butter, pumpkin, coconut milk, eggs, and vanilla until well blended.

3. In a small bowl, stir together the almond flour, erythritol, protein powder, baking powder, cinnamon, nutmeg, and cloves.

4. Add the dry ingredients to the wet ingredients and stir to combine.

5. Pour the mixture into the insert.

6. Cover and cook on low for 6 to 7 hours.

7. Serve warm.

VARIATION TIP: If you want to switch out the pumpkin, butternut or acorn squash make an absolutely lovely golden pudding and have only a few more grams of carbohydrates. If you want to use winter squash, use cooked as a substitute for canned.

BUTTERY COCONUT BREAD

MAKES 8 SLICES / PREP TIME: 10 MINUTES / COOK TIME: 3 TO 4 HOURS ON LOW

Warm bread is a real treat, especially with melted butter filling the nooks and crannies. This bread keeps well in the refrigerator and toasts beautifully. It pairs well with chicken breast for lunch or with peanut butter for breakfast.

1 TABLESPOON BUTTER, SOFTENED

6 LARGE EGGS

½ CUP COCONUT OIL, MELTED

1 TEASPOON PURE VANILLA EXTRACT

¼ TEASPOON LIQUID STEVIA

1 CUP ALMOND FLOUR

½ CUP COCONUT FLOUR

1 OUNCE PROTEIN POWDER

1 TEASPOON BAKING POWDER

1. Grease an 8-by-4-inch loaf pan with the butter.

2. In a medium bowl, whisk together the eggs, oil, vanilla, and stevia until well blended.

3. In a small bowl, stir together the almond flour, coconut flour, protein powder, and baking powder until mixed.

4. Add the dry ingredients to the wet ingredients and stir to combine.

5. Spoon the batter into the loaf pan and place the loaf pan on a rack in the slow cooker.

6. Cover and cook on low for 3 to 4 hours, until a knife inserted in the center comes out clean.

7. Cool the bread in the loaf pan for 15 minutes. Then remove the bread from the pan and place onto a wire rack to cool completely.

8. Store in a sealed container in the refrigerator for up to 1 week.

> **MAKE IT PALEO:** In the Paleo world, grass-fed butter is allowed according to some. If it is not on your acceptable-food list, you can omit the sweetener in this delightful bread to make it Paleo. Don't worry. The bread will still have a wonderful toasty flavor. If you don't eat butter, it can be replaced with coconut oil.

QUICK PREP

KETO QUOTIENT

MACRONUTRIENTS

72% FAT

17% PROTEIN

11% CARBS

PER SERVING

CALORIES: 336

TOTAL FAT: 28G

PROTEIN: 15G

TOTAL CARBS: 9G

FIBER: 6G

NET CARBS: 3G

CHOLESTEROL: 162MG

BREAKFAST SAUSAGE

SERVES 8 / PREP TIME: 10 MINUTES / COOK TIME: 3 HOURS ON LOW

**DAIRY-FREE
PALEO-FRIENDLY
QUICK PREP**

KETO QUOTIENT

MACRONUTRIENTS
72% FAT
26% PROTEIN
2% CARBS

PER SERVING
CALORIES: 341
TOTAL FAT: 27G
PROTEIN: 21G
TOTAL CARBS: 1G
FIBER: 0G
NET CARBS: 1G
CHOLESTEROL: 134MG

Processed sausages are not a recommended food on the keto diet unless they are organic and have no preservatives. Luckily, making your own is simple. You can create all kinds of different flavors from mild maple to spicy Italian depending on your preference. You can freeze the individually portioned cooked sausage in plastic bags and use them when you need them.

1 TABLESPOON EXTRA-VIRGIN OLIVE OIL

2 POUNDS GROUND PORK

2 EGGS

1 SWEET ONION, CHOPPED

½ CUP ALMOND FLOUR

2 TEASPOONS MINCED GARLIC

2 TEASPOONS DRIED OREGANO

1 TEASPOON DRIED THYME

1 TEASPOON FENNEL SEEDS

1 TEASPOON FRESHLY GROUND
    BLACK PEPPER

½ TEASPOON SALT

1. Lightly grease the insert of the slow cooker with the olive oil.

2. In a large bowl, stir together the pork, eggs, onion, almond flour, garlic, oregano, thyme, fennel seeds, pepper, and salt until well mixed.

3. Transfer the meat mixture to the slow cooker's insert and shape it into a loaf, leaving about ½ inch between the sides and meat.

4. Cover, and if your slow cooker has a temperature probe, insert it.

5. Cook on low until it reaches an internal temperature of 150°F, about 3 hours.

6. Slice in any way you prefer and serve.

ALLERGEN TIP: If tree nuts are an issue, simply leave out the almond flour and add 2 tablespoons of coconut flour instead as a binder. You do not have to add any extra eggs to compensate for the change.

HUEVOS RANCHEROS

SERVES 8 / PREP TIME: 10 MINUTES / COOK TIME: 3 HOURS ON LOW

You might be familiar with this popular dish often served with tortillas, but it is equally delicious as a stand-alone egg dish. For extra convenience, you can prepare the entire recipe the night before and store the insert in the refrigerator until the morning. Then, pop the insert into your slow cooker for a no-hassle breakfast.

1 TABLESPOON EXTRA-VIRGIN OLIVE OIL

10 EGGS

1 CUP HEAVY (WHIPPING) CREAM

1 CUP SHREDDED MONTEREY JACK
    CHEESE, DIVIDED

1 CUP PREPARED OR HOMEMADE SALSA

1 SCALLION, GREEN AND WHITE
    PARTS, CHOPPED

1 JALAPEÑO PEPPER, CHOPPED

½ TEASPOON CHILI POWDER

½ TEASPOON SALT

1 AVOCADO, CHOPPED, FOR GARNISH

1 TABLESPOON CHOPPED CILANTRO,
    FOR GARNISH

1. Lightly grease the insert of the slow cooker with the olive oil.

2. In a large bowl, whisk together the eggs, heavy cream, ½ cup of the cheese, salsa, scallion, jalapeño, chili powder, and salt. Pour the mixture into the insert and sprinkle the top with the remaining ½ cup of cheese.

3. Cover and cook until the eggs are firm, about 3 hours on low.

4. Let the eggs cool slightly, then cut into wedges and serve garnished with avocado and cilantro.

> **VARIATION TIP:** Jalapeño peppers are one of the more mild varieties of peppers. If you enjoy lots of heat in your food, substitute habanero or serrano peppers instead.

NUT-FREE

QUICK PREP

KETO QUOTIENT

MACRONUTRIENTS
77% FAT
17% PROTEIN
6% CARBS

PER SERVING
CALORIES: 302
TOTAL FAT: 26G
PROTEIN: 13G
TOTAL CARBS: 5G
FIBER: 2G
NET CARBS: 3G
CHOLESTEROL: 320MG

MEDITERRANEAN EGGS

SERVES 4 / PREP TIME: 10 MINUTES / COOK TIME: 5 TO 6 HOURS ON LOW

PALEO-FRIENDLY
QUICK PREP

KETO QUOTIENT

MACRONUTRIENTS
70% FAT
25% PROTEIN
5% CARBS

PER SERVING
CALORIES: 349
TOTAL FAT: 27G
PROTEIN: 23G
TOTAL CARBS: 5G
FIBER: 1G
NET CARBS: 4G
CHOLESTEROL: 641MG

If you are searching for a convenient meal for brunch or a late break-fast, look no farther than this vegetable-filled frittata. Pair this meal with crispy bacon or homemade sausage for guests. If you have left-overs, store individual portions in sealed plastic bags after they are completely cooled and enjoy them as a quick snack or light lunch, warm or cold.

1 TABLESPOON EXTRA-VIRGIN OLIVE OIL

12 EGGS

½ CUP COCONUT MILK

½ TEASPOON DRIED OREGANO

½ TEASPOON FRESHLY GROUND
   BLACK PEPPER

¼ TEASPOON SALT

2 CUPS CHOPPED SPINACH

1 TOMATO, CHOPPED

¼ CUP CHOPPED SWEET ONION

1 TEASPOON MINCED GARLIC

½ CUP CRUMBLED GOAT CHEESE

1. Lightly grease the insert of the slow cooker with the olive oil.

2. In a large bowl, whisk together the eggs, coconut milk, oregano, pepper, and salt, until well blended.

3. Add the spinach, tomato, onion, and garlic, and stir to combine.

4. Pour the egg mixture into the insert and top with the crumbled goat cheese.

5. Cover and cook on low 5 to 6 hours, until it is set like a quiche.

6. Serve warm.

VARIATION TIP: Any type of full-fat cheese would be delightful when com-bined with the fresh vegetables and herbs in this casserole. Feta, Cheddar, Swiss, and ricotta cheese are wonderful substitutes.

LAYERED EGG CASSEROLE

SERVES 12 / PREP TIME: 10 MINUTES / COOK TIME: 4 HOURS ON LOW

The colorful layers in this casserole look spectacular on your plate. The combination of sausage, fresh vegetables, and flavorful cheese is delicious warm or cold so any leftovers will be a welcome snack later in the day. Try yellow zucchini or orange peppers to change up the look of the dish.

1 TABLESPOON EXTRA-VIRGIN OLIVE OIL

1 POUND BREAKFAST SAUSAGE (PAGE 32)

1 ZUCCHINI, CHOPPED

1 RED BELL PEPPER, FINELY CHOPPED

½ SWEET ONION, CHOPPED

12 OUNCES SHREDDED CHEDDAR CHEESE

12 EGGS

1 CUP HEAVY (WHIPPING) CREAM

½ TEASPOON SALT

½ TEASPOON FRESHLY GROUND BLACK PEPPER

1. Lightly grease the insert of the slow cooker with the olive oil.

2. Arrange half of the sausage in the bottom of the insert. Top with half of the zucchini, pepper, and onion. Top the vegetables with half of the cheese. Repeat, creating another layer.

3. In a medium bowl, whisk together the eggs, heavy cream, salt, and pepper. Pour the egg mixture over the casserole.

4. Cover and cook on low for 4 hours.

5. Serve warm.

VARIATION TIP: Bacon or Canadian bacon could be substituted for the sausage in this dish. Whatever you use, make sure you use uncured meat that is brined without nitrites and nitrates.

QUICK PREP

KETO QUOTIENT

MACRONUTRIENTS
76% FAT
22% PROTEIN
2% CARBS

PER SERVING
CALORIES: 338
TOTAL FAT: 29G
PROTEIN: 18G
TOTAL CARBS: 2G
FIBER: 0G
NET CARBS: 2G
CHOLESTEROL: 285MG

SPANAKOPITA FRITTATA

SERVES 8 / PREP TIME: 10 MINUTES / 5 TO 6 HOURS ON LOW

NUT-FREE

QUICK PREP

KETO QUOTIENT

MACRONUTRIENTS
78% FAT
18% PROTEIN
4% CARBS

PER SERVING
CALORIES: 247
TOTAL FAT: 22G
PROTEIN: 11G
TOTAL CARBS: 2G
FIBER: 0G
NET CARBS: 2G
CHOLESTEROL: 364MG

Feta cheese tastes wonderful, and it is a great option if you are looking for something that tastes rich while you are on a diet. This green-flecked cheesy breakfast is inspired by the traditional Greek appetizer spanakopita and will surely become a family favorite.

1 TABLESPOON EXTRA-VIRGIN OLIVE OIL

12 EGGS

1 CUP HEAVY (WHIPPING) CREAM

2 TEASPOONS MINCED GARLIC

2 CUPS CHOPPED SPINACH

½ CUP FETA CHEESE

CHERRY TOMATOES, HALVED, FOR GARNISH (OPTIONAL)

YOGURT, FOR GARNISH (OPTIONAL)

PARSLEY, FOR GARNISH (OPTIONAL)

1. Lightly grease the insert of the slow cooker with the olive oil.

2. In a medium bowl, whisk together the eggs, heavy cream, garlic, spinach, and feta. Pour the mixture into the slow cooker.

3. Cover and cook on low 5 to 6 hours.

4. Serve topped with the the tomatoes, a dollop of yogurt, and parsley, if desired.

PRECOOKING TIP: Blanching the spinach in this recipe can create a smoother texture and a deeper green-colored frittata. Use 2 cups raw spinach and blanch for 2 minutes in boiling water. Make sure you squeeze out as much water as possible before adding the greens to the eggs.

CRUSTLESS WILD MUSHROOM-KALE QUICHE

SERVES 8 / PREP TIME: 10 MINUTES / COOK TIME: 5 TO 6 HOURS ON LOW

The earthy flavor and meaty texture of mushrooms pair beautifully with kale and sharp Swiss cheese in this quiche. There are many kinds of wild mushrooms to choose from that work in this dish, so get your favorite assortment of pretty fungi from your local super-market. If you use portobello mushrooms, scoop out the frilly dark gills underneath the cap before chopping them up. If you leave the gills, the eggs will turn an unpleasant gray color.

1 TABLESPOON EXTRA-VIRGIN OLIVE OIL

12 EGGS

1 CUP HEAVY (WHIPPING) CREAM

1 TABLESPOON CHOPPED FRESH THYME

1 TABLESPOON CHOPPED FRESH CHIVES

¼ TEASPOON FRESHLY GROUND
    BLACK PEPPER

⅛ TEASPOON SALT

2 CUPS COARSELY CHOPPED WILD
    MUSHROOMS (SHIITAKE, PORTOBELLO,
    OYSTER, ENOKI)

1 CUP CHOPPED KALE

1 CUP SHREDDED SWISS CHEESE

1. Lightly grease the insert of the slow cooker with the olive oil.

2. In a medium bowl, whisk together the eggs, heavy cream, thyme, chives, pepper, and salt. Stir in the mushrooms and kale. Pour the mixture into the slow cooker and top with the cheese.

3. Cover and cook on low 5 to 6 hours.

4. Serve warm.

> **MAKE IT PALEO:** Although the cheese adds a nice gooey topping to this dish, it also contributes several extra grams of fat and protein. You can omit it and swap the heavy cream for coconut milk to create a Paleo dish. The keto quotient will be low rather than medium.

BACON-AND-EGGS BREAKFAST CASSEROLE

SERVES 8 / PREP TIME: 15 MINUTES / COOK TIME: 5 TO 6 HOURS ON LOW

DAIRY-FREE
PALEO-FRIENDLY
QUICK PREP

KETO QUOTIENT

MACRONUTRIENTS
73% FAT
25% PROTEIN
2% CARBS

PER SERVING
CALORIES: 526
TOTAL FAT: 43G
PROTEIN: 32G
TOTAL CARBS: 3G
FIBER: 0G
NET CARBS: 3G
CHOLESTEROL: 421MG

Instead of your usual plate of bacon and eggs, imagine a convenient one-pot meal that you can cook while you are asleep. I always save bacon fat because it keeps well in the refrigerator—up to six months in a sealed jar—and you can use it for other recipes.

1 TABLESPOON BACON FAT OR EXTRA-VIRGIN OLIVE OIL

12 EGGS

1 CUP COCONUT MILK

1 POUND BACON, CHOPPED AND COOKED CRISP

½ SWEET ONION, CHOPPED

2 TEASPOONS MINCED GARLIC

¼ TEASPOON FRESHLY GROUND BLACK PEPPER

⅛ TEASPOON SALT

PINCH RED PEPPER FLAKES

1. Lightly grease the insert of the slow cooker with the bacon fat or olive oil.

2. In a medium bowl, whisk together the eggs, coconut milk, bacon, onion, garlic, pepper, salt, and red pepper flakes. Pour the mixture into the slow cooker.

3. Cover and cook on low for 5 to 6 hours.

4. Serve warm.

VARIATION TIP: If you do not need this tasty breakfast to be Paleo, try topping it with a cup of shredded sharp Cheddar cheese or crumbled creamy goat cheese.

VEGETABLE OMELET

SERVES 8 / PREP TIME: 15 MINUTES / COOK TIME: 4 TO 5 HOURS ON LOW

Omelets are usually cooked in a skillet, and the ingredients are tucked inside when the eggs are folded in half. This dish is not folded, but it is still crammed with hearty ingredients. If you want the broccoli and cauliflower to be softer in texture, you can blanch them in boiling water for two minutes before stirring them into the eggs.

1 TABLESPOON EXTRA-VIRGIN OLIVE OIL

10 EGGS

½ CUP HEAVY (WHIPPING) CREAM

1 TEASPOON MINCED GARLIC

¼ TEASPOON SALT

⅛ TEASPOON FRESHLY GROUND
    BLACK PEPPER

½ CUP CHOPPED CAULIFLOWER

½ CUP CHOPPED BROCCOLI

1 RED BELL PEPPER, CHOPPED

1 SCALLION, WHITE AND GREEN
    PARTS, CHOPPED

4 OUNCES GOAT CHEESE, CRUMBLED

2 TABLESPOONS CHOPPED PARSLEY,
    FOR GARNISH

1. Lightly grease the insert of the slow cooker with the olive oil.

2. In a medium bowl, whisk together the eggs, heavy cream, garlic, salt, and pepper. Stir in the cauliflower, broccoli, red bell pepper, and scallion. Pour the mixture into the slow cooker. Sprinkle the top with goat cheese.

3. Cover and cook on low for 4 to 5 hours.

4. Serve topped with the parsley.

> **ALLERGEN TIP:** If you are sensitive to milk, the heavy cream in the egg mixture can be changed to coconut milk or almond milk. You can omit or swap out the goat cheese as well.

NUT-FREE
QUICK PREP

KETO QUOTIENT

MACRONUTRIENTS
73% FAT
22% PROTEIN
5% CARBS

PER SERVING
CALORIES: 200
TOTAL FAT: 16G
PROTEIN: 11G
TOTAL CARBS: 2G
FIBER: 1G
NET CARBS: 1G
CHOLESTEROL: 291MG

SAUSAGE-STUFFED PEPPERS

SERVES 4 / PREP TIME: 15 MINUTES / COOK TIME: 4 TO 5 HOURS ON LOW

Tucking into this meal is sure to put you in a good mood. The peppers are tender, and when you cut through their skins, the perfectly cooked egg and gooey cheese filling spills out. Put them in the refrigerator to set the night before, and they will be ready to go in the morning.

1 TABLESPOON EXTRA-VIRGIN OLIVE OIL

4 BELL PEPPERS, TOPS CUT OFF AND SEEDS REMOVED

1 CUP BREAKFAST SAUSAGE (PAGE 32), CRUMBLED

6 EGGS

½ CUP COCONUT MILK

1 SCALLION, WHITE AND GREEN PARTS, CHOPPED

½ TEASPOON FRESHLY GROUND BLACK PEPPER

1 CUP SHREDDED CHEDDAR CHEESE

1. Line a slow cooker insert with foil and grease the foil with the olive oil.

2. Place the four peppers in the slow cooker and evenly fill them with the sausage crumbles.

3. In a medium bowl, whisk together the eggs, coconut milk, scallion, and pepper. Pour the egg mixture into the four peppers. Next, sprinkle the cheese over them.

4. Cook on low for 4 to 5 hours, until the eggs are set.

5. Serve warm.

> **VARIATION TIP:** Ground beef, chicken, or turkey can all stand in nicely for the sausage in the filling. If you use 80% lean protein, 20% fat products, then the keto macronutrient counts should not change dramatically.

DILL-ASPARAGUS BAKE

SERVES 8 / PREP TIME: 10 MINUTES / COOK TIME: 4 TO 5 HOURS ON LOW

Dill and asparagus are wonderful representations of spring on the culinary calendar. They are best in April, when they are tender and a glorious bright green in color. You want your asparagus to be about a pencil-width thick, avoid stems that look too much bigger than that. If your asparagus is a little thicker, chop about 1 inch off the bottom and use a vegetable peeler to pare the spears down.

1 TABLESPOON EXTRA-VIRGIN OLIVE OIL

10 EGGS

¾ CUP COCONUT MILK

½ TEASPOON SALT

¼ TEASPOON FRESHLY GROUND BLACK PEPPER

2 TEASPOONS CHOPPED FRESH DILL

2 CUPS CHOPPED ASPARAGUS SPEARS

1 CUP CHOPPED COOKED BACON

1. Lightly grease the insert of the slow cooker with the olive oil.

2. In a medium bowl, whisk together the eggs, coconut milk, salt, pepper, and dill. Stir in the asparagus and bacon. Pour the mixture into the slow cooker.

3. Cover and cook on low for 4 to 5 hours.

4. Serve warm.

PRECOOKING TIP: Raw asparagus works fine in this pretty spring-themed dish, but blanching the vegetable can help create a desired and uniform texture. Plunge the asparagus into boiling water for about 2 minutes, and then immediately run the spears under cold water. Dry them off with paper towels, chop them, and add them to the egg mixture.

DAIRY-FREE
PALEO-FRIENDLY
QUICK PREP

KETO QUOTIENT

MACRONUTRIENTS
75% FAT
20% PROTEIN
5% CARBS

PER SERVING
CALORIES: 225
TOTAL FAT: 18G
PROTEIN: 14G
TOTAL CARBS: 3G
FIBER: 1G
NET CARBS: 2G
CHOLESTEROL: 280MG

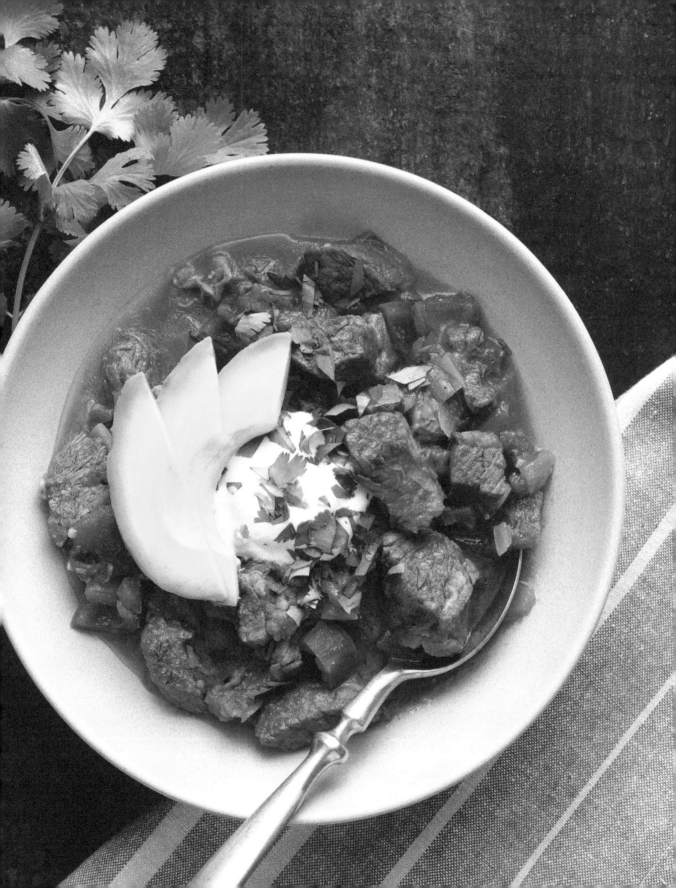

Chapter Four
SOUPS, STEWS & CHILI

◄—◄ SIMPLE TEXAS CHILI, PAGE 61

CHEDDAR CHEESE SOUP

SERVES 6 / PREP TIME: 15 MINUTES / COOK TIME: 6 HOURS ON LOW

QUICK PREP

KETO QUOTIENT

MACRONUTRIENTS
78% FAT
15% PROTEIN
7% CARBS

PER SERVING
CALORIES: 406
TOTAL FAT: 36G
PROTEIN: 15G
TOTAL CARBS: 7G
FIBER: 1G
NET CARBS: 6G
CHOLESTEROL: 88MG

There are various versions of cheese soup in countries across the world: *sopa de queso* in Spain, *Kassuppe* in Switzerland, and English Cheddar-beer soup, the basis for this beer-free British-style recipe. Look for orange Cheddar to get a rich flavor and pleasing color, although using white Cheddar is fine as well.

1 TABLESPOON BUTTER

5 CUPS CHICKEN BROTH

1 CUP COCONUT MILK

2 CELERY STALKS, CHOPPED

1 CARROT, CHOPPED

½ SWEET ONION, CHOPPED

PINCH CAYENNE PEPPER

8 OUNCES CREAM CHEESE, CUBED

2 CUPS SHREDDED CHEDDAR CHEESE

SALT, FOR SEASONING

FRESHLY GROUND BLACK PEPPER,
 FOR SEASONING

1 TABLESPOON CHOPPED FRESH THYME,
 FOR GARNISH

1. Lightly grease the insert of the slow cooker with the butter.

2. Place the broth, coconut milk, celery, carrot, onion, and cayenne pepper in the insert.

3. Cover and cook on low for 6 hours.

4. Stir in the cream cheese and Cheddar, then season with salt and pepper.

5. Serve topped with the thyme.

> **VARIATION TIP:** Cheddar adds a spectacularly rich flavor to this soup, but you can use any full-fat cheese with success. Swiss, Gouda, and provolone all create a luscious texture with subtly different tastes.

SAUSAGE-SAUERKRAUT SOUP

SERVES 6 / PREP TIME: 15 MINUTES / COOK TIME: 6 HOURS ON LOW

Hearty is the perfect word to describe this thick, Bavarian-inspired meal. Sauerkraut adds an enjoyable tanginess, which marries beautifully with savory sausage chunks. The mustard and sprinkling of caraway seeds give the dish a perfect combination of flavors. Try to source out German sausage that meets the keto parameters for a truly authentic experience.

1 TABLESPOON EXTRA-VIRGIN OLIVE OIL

6 CUPS BEEF BROTH

1 POUND ORGANIC SAUSAGE, COOKED AND SLICED

2 CUPS SAUERKRAUT

2 CELERY STALKS, CHOPPED

1 SWEET ONION, CHOPPED

2 TEASPOONS MINCED GARLIC

2 TABLESPOONS BUTTER

1 TABLESPOON HOT MUSTARD

½ TEASPOON CARAWAY SEEDS

½ CUP SOUR CREAM

2 TABLESPOONS CHOPPED FRESH PARSLEY, FOR GARNISH

1. Lightly grease the insert of the slow cooker with the olive oil.

2. Place the broth, sausage, sauerkraut, celery, onion, garlic, butter, mustard, and caraway seeds in the insert.

3. Cover and cook on low for 6 hours.

4. Stir in the sour cream.

5. Serve topped with the parsley.

> **ALLERGEN TIP:** If you are allergic to dairy, the sour cream can be omitted and the butter can be changed to coconut cream. This will change the keto quotient to low, but the macronutrient ratio will still be within the correct parameters.

NUT-FREE
QUICK PREP

KETO QUOTIENT

MACRONUTRIENTS
75% FAT
18% PROTEIN
7% CARBS

PER SERVING
CALORIES: 332
TOTAL FAT: 28G
PROTEIN: 15G
TOTAL CARBS: 6G
FIBER: 2G
NET CARBS: 4G
CHOLESTEROL: 69MG

CHEESY BACON-CAULIFLOWER SOUP

SERVES 6 / PREP TIME: 15 MINUTES / COOK TIME: 6 HOURS ON LOW

QUICK PREP

KETO QUOTIENT

MACRONUTRIENTS
70% FAT
25% PROTEIN
5% CARBS

PER SERVING
CALORIES: 540
TOTAL FAT: 44G
PROTEIN: 35G
TOTAL CARBS: 7G
FIBER: 1G
NET CARBS: 6G
CHOLESTEROL: 120MG

Creamy cauliflower soup topped with crispy bacon and rich cheese very popular at restaurants, and for good reason—the combination is spectacular. The bacon infuses every luscious spoonful in this version. However, you can save the bacon as a topping if you prefer that presentation of the dish.

1 TABLESPOON EXTRA-VIRGIN OLIVE OIL

4 CUPS CHICKEN BROTH

2 CUPS COCONUT MILK

2 CUPS CHOPPED COOKED CHICKEN

1 CUP CHOPPED COOKED BACON

2 CUPS CHOPPED CAULIFLOWER

1 SWEET ONION, CHOPPED

3 TEASPOONS MINCED GARLIC

½ CUP CREAM CHEESE, CUBED

2 CUPS SHREDDED CHEDDAR CHEESE

1. Lightly grease the insert of the slow cooker with the olive oil.

2. Place the broth, coconut milk, chicken, bacon, cauliflower, onion, and garlic in the insert.

3. Cover and cook on low for 6 hours.

4. Stir in the cream cheese and Cheddar and serve.

PRECOOKING TIP: If you only have raw chicken available, you can use that instead if you increase the cooking time to 7 to 8 hours. Just cut the raw chicken into ½-inch chunks first.

TURKEY-POTPIE SOUP

SERVES 8 / PREP TIME: 20 MINUTES / COOK TIME: 7 TO 8 HOURS ON LOW

This recipe is exactly like a turkey potpie, and all that is missing is the crust. If you prefer turkey thigh meat instead of breast, use that instead. To save some money, you can purchase a whole fresh turkey, separate the different sections into sealable freezer bags, and freeze them until you need them.

1 TABLESPOON EXTRA-VIRGIN OLIVE OIL

4 CUPS CHICKEN BROTH

½ POUND SKINLESS TURKEY BREAST, CUT INTO ½-INCH CHUNKS

2 CELERY STALKS, CHOPPED

1 CARROT, DICED

1 SWEET ONION, CHOPPED

2 TEASPOONS MINCED GARLIC

2 TEASPOONS CHOPPED FRESH THYME

1 CUP CREAM CHEESE, DICED

2 CUPS HEAVY (WHIPPING) CREAM

1 CUP GREEN BEANS, CUT INTO 1-INCH PIECES

SALT, FOR SEASONING

FRESHLY GROUND BLACK PEPPER, FOR SEASONING

1. Lightly grease the insert of the slow cooker with the olive oil.

2. Place the broth, turkey, celery, carrot, onion, garlic, and thyme in the insert.

3. Cover and cook on low for 7 to 8 hours.

4. Stir in the cream cheese, heavy cream, and green beans.

5. Season with salt and pepper and serve.

PRECOOKING TIP: The turkey can be browned in 2 tablespoons of olive oil in a skillet to create a lovely color and rich taste. This is not necessary, but it will cut down the cooking time by approximately 1 hour.

NUT-FREE

KETO QUOTIENT

MACRONUTRIENTS
74% FAT
20% PROTEIN
6% CARBS

PER SERVING
CALORIES: 415
TOTAL FAT: 35G
PROTEIN: 20G
TOTAL CARBS: 7G
FIBER: 2G
NET CARBS: 5G
CHOLESTEROL: 0MG

CHICKEN-NACHO SOUP

SERVES 8 / PREP TIME: 15 MINUTES / COOK TIME: 6 HOURS ON LOW

Nachos are an indulgence, usually consumed during a festive get-together with friends and family. With this dish, you can whip up a batch of soup in your slow cooker with all the same great flavors. Depending on your preference for heat and spice, adjust the seasonings and toppings to suit your palate. Be sure the taco seasoning mix you choose is keto friendly.

3 TABLESPOONS EXTRA-VIRGIN OLIVE OIL, DIVIDED

1 POUND GROUND CHICKEN

1 SWEET ONION, DICED

1 RED BELL PEPPER, CHOPPED

2 TEASPOONS MINCED GARLIC

2 TABLESPOONS TACO SEASONING

4 CUPS CHICKEN BROTH

2 CUPS COCONUT MILK

1 TOMATO, DICED

1 JALAPEÑO PEPPER, CHOPPED

2 CUPS SHREDDED CHEDDAR CHEESE

½ CUP SOUR CREAM, FOR GARNISH

1 SCALLION, WHITE AND GREEN PARTS, CHOPPED, FOR GARNISH

1. Lightly grease the insert of the slow cooker with 1 tablespoon of the olive oil.

2. In a large skillet over medium-high heat, heat the remaining 2 tablespoons of the olive oil. Add the chicken and sauté until it is cooked through, about 6 minutes.

3. Add the onion, red bell pepper, garlic, and taco seasoning, and sauté for an additional 3 minutes.

4. Transfer the chicken mixture to the insert, and stir in the broth, coconut milk, tomato, and jalapeño pepper.

5. Cover and cook on low for 6 hours.

6. Stir in the cheese.

7. Serve topped with the sour cream and scallion.

VARIATION TIP: Ground beef, pork, or turkey can all take the place of the chicken in this tempting soup. If you use ground beef, the macronutrient rations will change slightly with more fat and slightly less protein.

SPICED-PUMPKIN CHICKEN SOUP

SERVES 6 / PREP TIME: 15 MINUTES / COOK TIME: 6 HOURS ON LOW

Pumpkin is an incredibly versatile ingredient. In addition to starring in pumpkin pie, it is an appetizing choice for savory dishes such as stews and soups. Most grocery stores carry pumpkin, especially in the fall and winter, and it is often in the frozen food section. If you cannot find fresh pumpkin, you can use 1 (16-ounce) can puréed pumpkin for the soup instead. It might change the texture a little, but you will not be disappointed with the taste.

QUICK PREP

KETO QUOTIENT

MACRONUTRIENTS
74% FAT
15% PROTEIN
11% CARBS

PER SERVING
CALORIES: 389
TOTAL FAT: 32G
PROTEIN: 16G
TOTAL CARBS: 10G
FIBER: 5G
NET CARBS: 5G
CHOLESTEROL: 52MG

1 TABLESPOON EXTRA-VIRGIN OLIVE OIL

4 CUPS CHICKEN BROTH

2 CUPS COCONUT MILK

1 POUND PUMPKIN, DICED

½ SWEET ONION, CHOPPED

1 TABLESPOON GRATED FRESH GINGER

2 TEASPOONS MINCED GARLIC

½ TEASPOON GROUND CINNAMON

¼ TEASPOON GROUND NUTMEG

¼ TEASPOON FRESHLY GROUND
   BLACK PEPPER

¼ TEASPOON SALT

PINCH GROUND ALLSPICE

1 CUP HEAVY (WHIPPING) CREAM

2 CUPS CHOPPED COOKED CHICKEN

1. Lightly grease the insert of the slow cooker with the olive oil.

2. Place the broth, coconut milk, pumpkin, onion, ginger, garlic, cinnamon, nutmeg, pepper, salt, and allspice in the insert.

3. Cover and cook on low for 6 hours.

4. Using an immersion blender or a regular blender, purée the soup.

5. If you removed the soup from the insert to purée, add it back to the pot, and stir in the cream and chicken.

6. Keep heating the soup on low for 15 minutes to heat the chicken through, and then serve warm.

MAKE IT PALEO: Exchange the heavy cream with coconut milk. This will not change the keto ratios or the taste extensively.

FAUX LASAGNA SOUP

SERVES 6 / PREP TIME: 20 MINUTES / COOK TIME: 6 HOURS ON LOW

NUT-FREE

KETO QUOTIENT

MACRONUTRIENTS
70% FAT
25% PROTEIN
5% CARBS

PER SERVING
CALORIES: 472
TOTAL FAT: 36G
PROTEIN: 30G
TOTAL CARBS: 9G
FIBER: 3G
NET CARBS: 6G
CHOLESTEROL: 111MG

The only traditional lasagna ingredient missing from this substantial meal is the noodles, but don't worry—you won't miss them. The soup broth is cheesy and has a marvelous beef taste from slow cooking, so make sure not to waste any. You can add red bell pepper or mushrooms to the recipe for more texture and color.

3 TABLESPOONS EXTRA-VIRGIN OLIVE OIL, DIVIDED

1 POUND GROUND BEEF

½ SWEET ONION, CHOPPED

2 TEASPOONS MINCED GARLIC

4 CUPS BEEF BROTH

1 (28-OUNCE) CAN DICED TOMATOES, UNDRAINED

1 ZUCCHINI, DICED

1½ TABLESPOONS DRIED BASIL

2 TEASPOONS DRIED OREGANO

4 OUNCES CREAM CHEESE

1 CUP SHREDDED MOZZARELLA

1. Lightly grease the insert of the slow cooker with 1 tablespoon of the olive oil.

2. In a large skillet over medium-high heat, heat the remaining 2 tablespoons of the olive oil. Add the ground beef and sauté until it is cooked through, about 6 minutes.

3. Add the onion and garlic and sauté for an additional 3 minutes.

4. Transfer the meat mixture to the insert.

5. Stir in the broth, tomatoes, zucchini, basil, and oregano.

6. Cover and cook on low for 6 hours.

7. Stir in the cream cheese and mozzarella and serve.

VARIATION TIP: A good quality low-carb marinara sauce, such as Simple Marinara Sauce (page 165), can be used in place of the diced tomatoes. Just use 2 cups of sauce for a thicker soup.

CHICKEN-BACON SOUP

SERVES 8 / PREP TIME: 15 MINUTES / COOK TIME: 8 HOURS ON LOW

Crispy bacon, cheesy broth, and hearty chunks of chicken and vegetables combine to create a thick, scrumptious soup that can serve as a light meal rather than an appetizer. This dish is a wonderful way to use up leftover roast chicken, which can also be conveniently cooked in a slow cooker. Strip off the meat from the chicken carcass and store it in a sealed bag in the refrigerator or freezer until you are ready to use it for this recipe.

1 TABLESPOON EXTRA-VIRGIN OLIVE OIL

6 CUPS CHICKEN BROTH

3 CUPS COOKED CHICKEN, CHOPPED

1 SWEET ONION, CHOPPED

2 CELERY STALKS, CHOPPED

1 CARROT, DICED

2 TEASPOONS MINCED GARLIC

1½ CUPS HEAVY (WHIPPING) CREAM

1 CUP CREAM CHEESE

1 CUP COOKED CHOPPED BACON

1 TABLESPOON CHOPPED FRESH PARSLEY, FOR GARNISH

1. Lightly grease the insert of the slow cooker with the olive oil.
2. Add the broth, chicken, onion, celery, carrot, and garlic.
3. Cover and cook on low for 8 hours.
4. Stir in the heavy cream, cream cheese, and bacon.
5. Serve topped with the parsley.

> **MAKE IT PALEO:** The heavy cream and cream cheese can be replaced by 2 cups of coconut milk, including the coconut cream at the top of the can. This will change the flavor slightly, but the bacon topping combines well with these ingredients too.

NUT-FREE
ALLERGEN-FREE
QUICK PREP

KETO QUOTIENT

MACRONUTRIENTS
70% FAT
20% PROTEIN
10% CARBS

PER SERVING
CALORIES: 488
TOTAL FAT: 37G
PROTEIN: 27G
TOTAL CARBS: 11G
FIBER: 1G
NET CARBS: 10G
CHOLESTEROL: 156MG

HOMEMADE SAUSAGE SOUP

SERVES 6 / PREP TIME: 15 MINUTES / COOK TIME: 6 HOURS ON LOW

DAIRY-FREE
NUT-FREE
ALLERGEN-FREE
PALEO-FRIENDLY
QUICK PREP

KETO QUOTIENT

MACRONUTRIENTS
73% FAT
22% PROTEIN
5% CARBS

PER SERVING
CALORIES: 383
TOTAL FAT: 31G
PROTEIN: 21G
TOTAL CARBS: 5G
FIBER: 1G
NET CARBS: 4G
CHOLESTEROL: 71MG

Sausage meat can be bought without the casings in the grocery store, or you can split them yourself, but you can also use Breakfast Sausage (page 32) to make tasty soup for a hearty lunch or dinner. This is a great base recipe for many variations. Add whatever you love: cheese, chopped cauliflower, or chicken.

3 TABLESPOONS OLIVE OIL, DIVIDED

1½ POUNDS SAUSAGE, WITHOUT CASING

6 CUPS CHICKEN BROTH

2 CELERY STALKS, CHOPPED

1 CARROT, DICED

1 LEEK, THOROUGHLY CLEANED AND CHOPPED

2 TEASPOONS MINCED GARLIC

2 CUPS CHOPPED KALE

1 TABLESPOON CHOPPED FRESH PARSLEY, FOR GARNISH

1. Lightly grease the insert of the slow cooker with 1 tablespoon of the olive oil.

2. In a large skillet over medium-high heat, heat the remaining 2 tablespoons of the olive oil. Add the sausage and sauté until it is cooked through, about 7 minutes.

3. Transfer the sausage to the insert, and stir in the broth, celery, carrot, leek, and garlic.

4. Cover and cook on low for 6 hours.

5. Stir in the kale.

6. Serve topped with the parsley.

> **VARIATION TIP:** Any dark, leafy green would be fabulous in this hearty soup, so try whatever is in your refrigerator or garden. Spinach, Swiss chard, collard greens, or beet greens all have comparable nutrition profiles and add similar amounts of protein and carbs to the dish.

CHEESEBURGER SOUP

SERVES 8 / PREP TIME: 15 MINUTES / COOK TIME: 6 HOURS ON LOW

Cheeseburger soup is a classic family favorite in many homes, and it can be made perfectly in a slow cooker with very little prep time. If you have never had this dish, the taste of your favorite sandwich in a bowl is a wonderful surprise. Top it with a little diced tomato and chopped pickles for a real burger experience.

3 TABLESPOONS OLIVE OIL, DIVIDED

1 POUND GROUND BEEF

1 SWEET ONION, CHOPPED

2 TEASPOONS MINCED GARLIC

6 CUPS BEEF BROTH

1 (28-OUNCE) CAN DICED TOMATOES

2 CELERY STALKS, CHOPPED

1 CARROT, CHOPPED

1 CUP HEAVY (WHIPPING) CREAM

2 CUPS SHREDDED CHEDDAR CHEESE

½ TEASPOON FRESHLY GROUND BLACK PEPPER

1 SCALLION, WHITE AND GREEN PARTS, CHOPPED, FOR GARNISH

1. Lightly grease the insert of the slow cooker with 1 tablespoon of the olive oil.

2. In a large skillet over medium-high heat, heat the remaining 2 tablespoons of the olive oil. Add the ground beef and sauté until it is cooked through, about 6 minutes.

3. Add the onion and garlic and sauté for an additional 3 minutes.

4. Transfer the beef mixture to the insert, and stir in the broth, tomatoes, celery, and carrot.

5. Cover and cook on low for 6 hours.

6. Stir in the heavy cream, cheese, and pepper.

7. Serve hot, topped with the scallion.

MAKE IT PALEO: Hamburger soup can be just as delicious as cheeseburger soup, although you will lose some of the fat grams. Instead of the cheese, add a cup of crispy cooked bacon and change the cream to coconut milk.

JAMBALAYA SOUP

SERVES 8 / PREP TIME: 15 MINUTES / COOK TIME: 6 TO 7 HOURS ON LOW

NUT-FREE
QUICK PREP

KETO QUOTIENT

MACRONUTRIENTS
70% FAT
25% PROTEIN
5% CARBS

PER SERVING
CALORIES: 400
TOTAL FAT: 31G
PROTEIN: 24G
TOTAL CARBS: 9G
FIBER: 4G
NET CARBS: 5G
CHOLESTEROL: 123MG

Jambalaya is a traditional Cajun and Creole spicy rice dish from Louisiana, and is influenced by both Spanish and French cuisine. This recipe is based on the Cajun version, and is bursting with poultry, sausage, and shrimp. The flavors and textures work well as a soup, and it is just as filling as its rice-based counterpart. If you do not have time at the end of the cooking process to wait 30 minutes for raw shrimp to cook, you can use small precooked shrimp instead. Let them heat up in the steaming broth while you set your table.

1 TABLESPOON EXTRA-VIRGIN OLIVE OIL

6 CUPS CHICKEN BROTH

1 (28-OUNCE) CAN DICED TOMATOES

1 POUND SPICY ORGANIC SAUSAGE, SLICED

1 CUP CHOPPED COOKED CHICKEN

1 RED BELL PEPPER, CHOPPED

½ SWEET ONION, CHOPPED

1 JALAPEÑO PEPPER, CHOPPED

2 TEASPOONS MINCED GARLIC

3 TABLESPOONS CAJUN SEASONING

½ POUND MEDIUM SHRIMP, PEELED, DEVEINED, AND CHOPPED

½ CUP SOUR CREAM, FOR GARNISH

1 AVOCADO, DICED, FOR GARNISH

2 TABLESPOONS CHOPPED CILANTRO, FOR GARNISH

1. Lightly grease the insert of the slow cooker with the olive oil.

2. Add the broth, tomatoes, sausage, chicken, red bell pepper, onion, jalapeño pepper, garlic, and Cajun seasoning.

3. Cover and cook on low for 6 to 7 hours.

4. Stir in the shrimp and leave on low for 30 minutes, or until the shrimp are cooked through.

5. Serve topped with the sour cream, avocado, and cilantro.

ALLERGEN TIP: Jambalaya traditionally features shrimp in the ingredient list, but you can leave this popular shellfish out if you have an allergy. The sour cream can be replaced with coconut cream to eliminate the dairy as well.

SIMPLE CHICKEN-VEGETABLE SOUP

SERVES 6 / PREP TIME: 15 MINUTES / COOK TIME: 7 TO 8 HOURS ON LOW

Who doesn't crave chicken soup when they are feeling under the weather and want something comforting and homey? When you know you have a long day ahead of you or you feel a cold coming on, throw together this mouthwatering creation to enjoy when you get home and curl up on the couch. It is even better the second day, so take a container to work as a wholesome meal for lunch.

1 TABLESPOON EXTRA-VIRGIN OLIVE OIL

4 CUPS CHICKEN BROTH

2 CUPS COCONUT MILK

2 CUPS DICED CHICKEN BREAST

½ SWEET ONION, CHOPPED

2 CELERY STALKS, CHOPPED

1 CARROT, DICED

½ CUP CHOPPED CAULIFLOWER

2 TEASPOONS MINCED GARLIC

1 TEASPOON CHOPPED THYME

1 TEASPOON CHOPPED OREGANO

¼ TEASPOON FRESHLY GROUND BLACK PEPPER

1. Lightly grease the insert of the slow cooker with the olive oil.

2. Add the broth, coconut milk, chicken, onion, celery, carrot, cauliflower, garlic, thyme, oregano, and pepper.

3. Cover and cook on low for 7 to 8 hours.

4. Serve warm.

> **PRECOOKING TIP:** Sautéing the raw chicken chunks in either coconut oil or olive oil can be a useful step to seal in some of the juices in the chicken. Slow-cooking proteins can sometimes produce a dry result, so this step can create a better dish.

DAIRY-FREE
ALLERGEN-FREE
PALEO-FRIENDLY
QUICK PREP

KETO QUOTIENT

MACRONUTRIENTS
75% FAT
19% PROTEIN
6% CARBS

PER SERVING
CALORIES: 299
TOTAL FAT: 25G
PROTEIN: 14G
TOTAL CARBS: 8G
FIBER: 3G
NET CARBS: 5G
CHOLESTEROL: 25MG

BEEF STEW

SERVES 6 / PREP TIME: 15 MINUTES / COOK TIME: 8 HOURS ON LOW

Tender chunks of beef in rich gravy are perfect when served over fluffy mashed cauliflower at the end of a long day. The scent of this stew cooking when you open your door will draw you to the kitchen before you have taken your coat off. This recipe tastes even better the next day and freezes beautifully, so it is very convenient for meal planning.

3 TABLESPOONS EXTRA-VIRGIN OLIVE OIL, DIVIDED

1 (2-POUND) BEEF CHUCK ROAST, CUT INTO 1-INCH CHUNKS

½ TEASPOON SALT

¼ TEASPOON FRESHLY GROUND BLACK PEPPER

2 CUPS BEEF BROTH

1 CUP DICED TOMATOES

¼ CUP APPLE CIDER VINEGAR

1½ CUPS CUBED PUMPKIN, CUT INTO 1-INCH CHUNKS

½ SWEET ONION, CHOPPED

2 TEASPOONS MINCED GARLIC

1 TEASPOON DRIED THYME

1 TABLESPOON CHOPPED FRESH PARSLEY, FOR GARNISH

1. Lightly grease the insert of the slow cooker with 1 tablespoon of the olive oil.

2. Lightly season the beef chucks with salt and pepper.

3. In a large skillet over medium-high heat, heat the remaining 2 tablespoons of the olive oil. Add the beef and brown on all sides, about 7 minutes.

4. Transfer the beef to the insert and stir in the broth, tomatoes, apple cider vinegar, pumpkin, onion, garlic, and thyme.

5. Cover and cook on low heat for about 8 hours, until the beef is very tender.

6. Serve topped with the parsley.

VARIATION TIP: This recipe would be enhanced by ½ cup dry red wine added in for ½ cup of the beef broth. Red wine adds depth to the flavor and, in this amount, less than ½ gram of carbs per serving.

CREAMY CHICKEN STEW

SERVES 6 / PREP TIME: 20 MINUTES / COOK TIME: 6 HOURS ON LOW

Chicken thighs are often overlooked at the meat counter because breasts are considered to be healthier. However, thighs are juicier, and have more flavor than the white meat components of the bird. They are fabulous when prepared in a slow cooker, adding richness to the creamy sauce in this recipe.

3 TABLESPOONS EXTRA-VIRGIN OLIVE OIL, DIVIDED

1 POUND BONELESS CHICKEN THIGHS, DICED INTO 1½-INCH PIECES

½ SWEET ONION, CHOPPED

2 TEASPOONS MINCED GARLIC

2 CUPS CHICKEN BROTH

2 CELERY STALKS, DICED

1 CARROT, DICED

1 TEASPOON DRIED THYME

1 CUP SHREDDED KALE

1 CUP COCONUT CREAM

SALT, FOR SEASONING

FRESHLY GROUND BLACK PEPPER, FOR SEASONING

1. Lightly grease the insert of the slow cooker with 1 tablespoon of the olive oil.

2. In a large skillet over medium-high heat, heat the remaining 2 tablespoons of the olive oil. Add the chicken and sauté until it is just cooked through, about 7 minutes.

3. Add the onion and garlic and sauté for an additional 3 minutes.

4. Transfer the chicken mixture to the insert, and stir in the broth, celery, carrot, and thyme.

5. Cover and cook on low for 6 hours.

6. Stir in the kale and coconut cream.

7. Season with salt and pepper, and serve warm.

> **PRECOOKING TIP:** If the chicken thighs you are using for this recipe do not have the skin on them, you can skip the searing step and add the chicken pieces directly into the insert along with the raw onion and garlic. Increase the cooking time to 7 to 8 hours to make up for not precooking the poultry.

**DAIRY-FREE
ALLERGEN-FREE
PALEO-FRIENDLY**

KETO QUOTIENT

MACRONUTRIENTS
70% FAT
25% PROTEIN
5% CARBS

PER SERVING
CALORIES: 276
TOTAL FAT: 22G
PROTEIN: 17G
TOTAL CARBS: 6G
FIBER: 2G
NET CARBS: 4G
CHOLESTEROL: 0MG

CURRIED VEGETABLE STEW

SERVES 6 / PREP TIME: 15 MINUTES / COOK TIME: 7 TO 8 HOURS ON LOW

Vegetables come in a fabulous assortment of tastes and interesting textures, so try your favorites to create a pleasing combination in this stew. Most vegetables are budget friendly, especially when in season, so this entire pot will not set you back too much. Vegetables such as zucchini and cauliflower soak up the flavor of the added spices and herbs. The broth is a beautiful combination of curry and fresh ginger complimented by the coconut milk base.

1 TABLESPOON EXTRA-VIRGIN OLIVE OIL

4 CUPS COCONUT MILK

1 CUP DICED PUMPKIN

1 CUP CAULIFLOWER FLORETS

1 RED BELL PEPPER, DICED

1 ZUCCHINI, DICED

1 SWEET ONION, CHOPPED

2 TEASPOONS GRATED FRESH GINGER

2 TEASPOONS MINCED GARLIC

1 TABLESPOON CURRY POWDER

2 CUPS SHREDDED SPINACH

1 AVOCADO, DICED, FOR GARNISH

1. Lightly grease the insert of the slow cooker with the olive oil.
2. Add the coconut milk, pumpkin, cauliflower, bell pepper, zucchini, onion, ginger, garlic, and curry powder.
3. Cover and cook on low for 7 to 8 hours.
4. Stir in the spinach.
5. Garnish each bowl with a spoonful of avocado and serve.

VARIATION TIP: Curry combines well with almost any ingredient so if you want to change the vegetables in this dish or add meat, go right ahead. Butternut squash, broccoli, okra, bok choy, and carrots could all be delicious in this creamy, spicy sauce.

TURKEY-VEGETABLE STEW

SERVES 6 / PREP TIME: 20 MINUTES / COOK TIME: 7 TO 8 HOURS ON LOW

While chicken and turkey stews are very similar, turkey has a more distinctive and stronger taste than chicken. It allows you to use more assertive seasonings, and the scent of this stew in the slow cooker will remind you of Thanksgiving or Christmas dinner.

3 TABLESPOONS EXTRA-VIRGIN OLIVE OIL, DIVIDED

1 POUND BONELESS TURKEY BREAST, CUT INTO 1-INCH PIECES

1 LEEK, THOROUGHLY CLEANED AND SLICED

2 TEASPOONS MINCED GARLIC

2 CUPS CHICKEN BROTH

1 CUP COCONUT MILK

2 CELERY STALKS, CHOPPED

2 CUPS DICED PUMPKIN

1 CARROT, DICED

2 TEASPOONS CHOPPED THYME

SALT, FOR SEASONING

FRESHLY GROUND BLACK PEPPER, FOR SEASONING

1 SCALLION, WHITE AND GREEN PARTS, CHOPPED, FOR GARNISH

1. Lightly grease the insert of the slow cooker with 1 tablespoon of the olive oil.

2. In a large skillet over medium-high heat, heat the remaining 2 tablespoons of the olive oil. Add the turkey and sauté until browned, about 5 minutes.

3. Add the leek and garlic and sauté for an additional 3 minutes.

4. Transfer the turkey mixture to the insert and stir in the broth, coconut milk, celery, pumpkin, carrot, and thyme.

5. Cover and cook on low for 7 to 8 hours.

6. Season with salt and pepper.

7. Serve topped with the scallion.

> **VARIATION TIP:** Stew is the perfect way to use up meats and vegetables in your refrigerator, so try beef, chicken, or pork if you are feeling adventurous. This substitution will not affect the cooking time or keto ratios dramatically.

DAIRY-FREE
ALLERGEN-FREE
PALEO-FRIENDLY

KETO QUOTIENT

MACRONUTRIENTS
70% FAT
23% PROTEIN
7% CARBS

PER SERVING
CALORIES: 356
TOTAL FAT: 27G
PROTEIN: 21G
TOTAL CARBS: 11G
FIBER: 4G
NET CARBS: 7G
CHOLESTEROL: 58MG

CHIPOTLE CHICKEN CHILI

SERVES 6 / PREP TIME: 20 MINUTES / COOK TIME: 7 TO 8 HOURS ON LOW

NUT-FREE

KETO QUOTIENT

MACRONUTRIENTS
70% FAT
24% PROTEIN
6% CARBS

PER SERVING
CALORIES: 390
TOTAL FAT: 30G
PROTEIN: 22G
TOTAL CARBS: 14G
FIBER: 5G
NET CARBS: 9G
CHOLESTEROL: 102MG

Chili is one of the easiest slow-cooker meals to make because the longer you cook it, the deeper and more complex the flavors will be. Chipotle chili powder can be found in the spice section of the supermarket. The unique smoky heat this spice adds to the chili is unforgettable and simply dances on your tongue. Do not use too much, though, because it does pack some substantial heat.

3 TABLESPOONS EXTRA-VIRGIN OLIVE OIL, DIVIDED

1 POUND GROUND CHICKEN

½ SWEET ONION, CHOPPED

2 TEASPOONS MINCED GARLIC

1 (28-OUNCE) CAN DICED TOMATOES

1 CUP CHICKEN BROTH

1 CUP DICED PUMPKIN

1 GREEN BELL PEPPER, DICED

3 TABLESPOONS CHILI POWDER

1 TEASPOON CHIPOTLE CHILI POWDER

1 CUP SOUR CREAM, FOR GARNISH

1 CUP SHREDDED CHEDDAR CHEESE, FOR GARNISH

1. Lightly grease the insert of the slow cooker with 1 tablespoon of the olive oil.

2. In a large skillet over medium-high heat, heat the remaining 2 tablespoons of the olive oil. Add the chicken and sauté until it is cooked through, about 6 minutes.

3. Add the onion and garlic and sauté for an additional 3 minutes.

4. Transfer the chicken mixture to the insert and stir in the tomatoes, broth, pumpkin, bell pepper, chili powder, and chipotle chili powder.

5. Cover and cook on low for 7 to 8 hours.

6. Serve topped with the sour cream and cheese.

VARIATION TIP: To save some prep time, you can use whole chicken breasts cut into ½-inch chunks instead of ground chicken. Just add the chicken chunks, onion, and garlic to the slow cooker with the tomatoes, broth, and other ingredients.

SIMPLE TEXAS CHILI

SERVES 4 / PREP TIME: 20 MINUTES / COOK TIME: 7 TO 8 HOURS ON LOW

Entire events are planned around the cooking and eating of chili. This recipe uses beef chunks rather than ground beef. The chunks become fork tender and sometimes break down into shreds that soak up the spicy sauce. Adjust the seasonings to create hotter or milder versions of the chili. This dish is even better served the next day, after the flavors have combined further.

NUT-FREE

KETO QUOTIENT

MACRONUTRIENTS
70% FAT
21% PROTEIN
9% CARBS

PER SERVING
CALORIES: 487
TOTAL FAT: 38G
PROTEIN: 26G
TOTAL CARBS: 17G
FIBER: 7G
NET CARBS: 10G
CHOLESTEROL: 84MG

¼ CUP EXTRA-VIRGIN OLIVE OIL

1½ POUNDS BEEF SIRLOIN, CUT INTO 1-INCH CHUNKS

1 SWEET ONION, CHOPPED

2 GREEN BELL PEPPERS, CHOPPED

1 JALAPEÑO PEPPER, SEEDED, FINELY CHOPPED

2 TEASPOONS MINCED GARLIC

1 (28-OUNCE) CAN DICED TOMATOES

1 CUP BEEF BROTH

3 TABLESPOONS CHILI POWDER

½ TEASPOON GROUND CUMIN

¼ TEASPOON GROUND CORIANDER

1 CUP SOUR CREAM, FOR GARNISH

1 AVOCADO, DICED, FOR GARNISH

1 TABLESPOON CILANTRO, CHOPPED, FOR GARNISH

1. Lightly grease the insert of the slow cooker with 1 tablespoon of the olive oil.

2. In a large skillet over medium-high heat, heat the remaining 2 tablespoons of the olive oil. Add the beef and sauté until it is cooked through, about 8 minutes.

3. Add the onion, bell peppers, jalapeño pepper, and garlic, and sauté for an additional 4 minutes.

4. Transfer the beef mixture to the insert and stir in the tomatoes, broth, chili powder, cumin, and coriander.

5. Cover and cook on low for 7 to 8 hours.

6. Serve topped with the sour cream, avocado, and cilantro.

> **MAKE IT PALEO:** Omit the sour cream topping on the chili if you want a Paleo dish. This will decrease the keto quotient and macronutrient ratios, so add a couple of fat bombs as snacks to level out your daily totals. Fat bombs are keto snacks made with fat-heavy ingredients such as bacon fat, cream cheese, and other luscious choices.

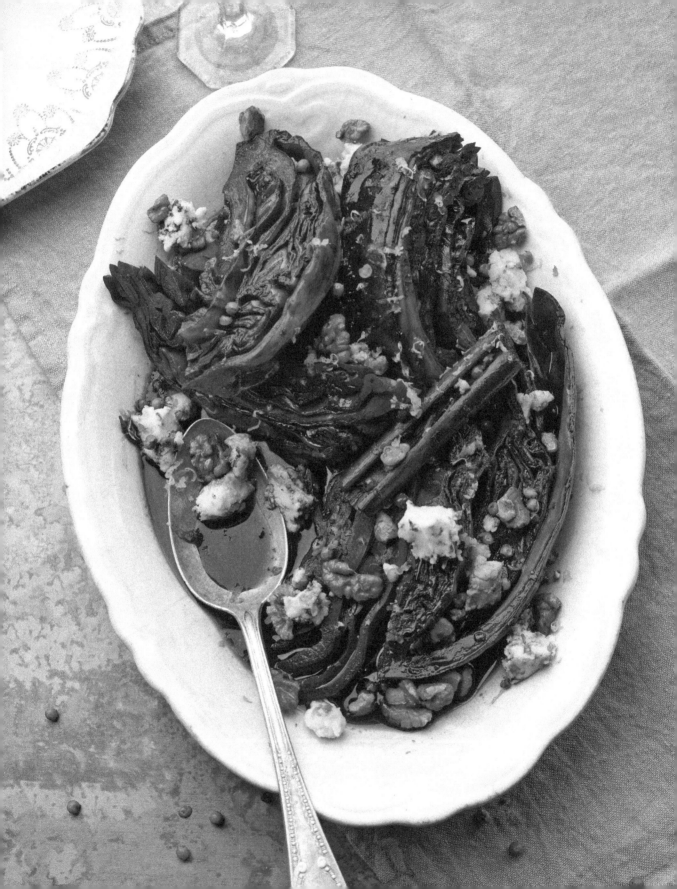

Chapter Five

VEGETABLES & VEGETARIAN DISHES

SWEET-BRAISED RED CABBAGE, PAGE 73

CREAMED VEGETABLES

SERVES 6 / PREP TIME: 15 MINUTES / COOK TIME: 6 HOURS ON LOW

The beauty of this dish is its flexibility. The vegetables in this dish can reflect the current offerings of your farmers' market or supermarket. Be inspired by what's in season. There is a broad range of vegetables allowed on the keto diet, so create a new combination every time you make this recipe.

1 TABLESPOON EXTRA-VIRGIN OLIVE OIL

½ HEAD CAULIFLOWER, CUT INTO SMALL FLORETS

2 CUPS GREEN BEANS, CUT INTO 2-INCH PIECES

1 CUP ASPARAGUS SPEARS, CUT INTO 2-INCH PIECES

½ CUP SOUR CREAM

½ CUP SHREDDED CHEDDAR CHEESE

½ CUP SHREDDED SWISS CHEESE

3 TABLESPOONS BUTTER

¼ CUP WATER

1 TEASPOON GROUND NUTMEG

PINCH FRESHLY GROUND BLACK PEPPER, FOR SEASONING

1. Lightly grease the insert of the slow cooker with the olive oil.

2. Add the cauliflower, green beans, asparagus, sour cream, Cheddar cheese, Swiss cheese, butter, water, nutmeg, and pepper to the insert.

3. Cover and cook on low for 6 hours.

4. Serve warm.

VARIATION TIP: Be creative with your vegetable choices, as most will taste fabulous with the cheese and butter in this recipe. Try broccoli, carrots, bok choy, and red bell peppers for interesting variations.

CARROT-PUMPKIN PUDDING

SERVES 6 / PREP TIME: 15 MINUTES / COOK TIME: 6 HOURS ON LOW

This is the perfect side dish. It is sweet and has a lovely creamy texture that pairs well with any type of protein. You might even be tempted to eat the pudding as a snack or for breakfast. To boost the protein ratio of the dish, simply add a scoop of plain protein powder.

1 TABLESPOON EXTRA-VIRGIN OLIVE OIL OR
GHEE (PAGE 158)

2 CUPS FINELY SHREDDED CARROTS

2 CUPS PURÉED PUMPKIN

½ SWEET ONION, FINELY CHOPPED

1 CUP HEAVY (WHIPPING) CREAM

½ CUP CREAM CHEESE, SOFTENED

2 EGGS

1 TABLESPOON GRANULATED ERYTHRITOL

1 TEASPOON GROUND NUTMEG

½ TEASPOON SALT

¼ CUP PUMPKIN SEEDS, FOR GARNISH

1. Lightly grease the insert of the slow cooker with the olive oil or ghee.

2. In a large bowl, whisk together the carrots, pumpkin, onion, heavy cream, cream cheese, eggs, erythritol, nutmeg, and salt.

3. Cover and cook on low for 6 hours.

4. Serve warm, topped with the pumpkin seeds.

> **ALLERGEN TIP:** If you have an issue with eggs, you can use a "faux" egg as a binder in this recipe. Stir together 2 tablespoons of ground flaxseed with 6 tablespoons of water and let the mixture stand in the refrigerator for 15 minutes before adding it.

NUT-FREE
QUICK PREP

KETO QUOTIENT

MACRONUTRIENTS
74% FAT
10% PROTEIN
16% CARBS

PER SERVING
CALORIES: 239
TOTAL FAT: 19G
PROTEIN: 6G
TOTAL CARBS: 11G
FIBER: 4G
NET CARBS: 7G
CHOLESTEROL: 103MG

CREAMY BROCCOLI CASSEROLE

SERVES 6 / PREP TIME: 15 MINUTES / COOK TIME: 6 HOURS ON LOW

In the 1980s, a casserole called Chicken Divan was very popular, despite being high in fat. That decadent dish inspired this Creamy Broccoli Casserole. There is cauliflower in the casserole as well, but you can leave it out if you want a pure broccoli creation.

1 TABLESPOON EXTRA-VIRGIN OLIVE OIL

1 POUND BROCCOLI, CUT INTO FLORETS

1 POUND CAULIFLOWER, CUT INTO FLORETS

¼ CUP ALMOND FLOUR

2 CUPS COCONUT MILK

½ TEASPOON GROUND NUTMEG

PINCH FRESHLY GROUND BLACK PEPPER

1½ CUPS SHREDDED GOUDA CHEESE, DIVIDED

1. Lightly grease the insert of the slow cooker with the olive oil.

2. Place the broccoli and cauliflower in the insert.

3. In a small bowl, stir together the almond flour, coconut milk, nutmeg, pepper, and 1 cup of the cheese.

4. Pour the coconut milk mixture over the vegetables and top the casserole with the remaining ½ cup of the cheese.

5. Cover and cook on low for 6 hours.

6. Serve warm.

ALLERGEN TIP: The almond flour can be replaced with coconut flour if tree nuts pose a problem for you. Just use 1 tablespoon of the coconut flour as the thickening and binding agent in this recipe.

CAULIFLOWER-PECAN CASSEROLE

SERVES 6 / PREP TIME: 15 MINUTES / COOK TIME: 6 HOURS ON LOW

Cauliflower is a well-liked cruciferous vegetable. It is a spectacular choice for a side dish because it melds so well with so many flavors and cuisines. The mild-tasting cauliflower serves as the base in this dish without adding many carbs and lets the rich flavor of the bacon, pecans, and eggs shine through. Don't forget the lemon juice because it brightens the taste of the whole combination.

1 TABLESPOON EXTRA-VIRGIN OLIVE OIL

2 POUNDS CAULIFLOWER FLORETS

10 BACON SLICES, COOKED AND CHOPPED

1 CUP CHOPPED PECANS

4 GARLIC CLOVES, SLICED

½ TEASPOON SALT

½ TEASPOON FRESHLY GROUND BLACK PEPPER

2 TABLESPOONS FRESHLY SQUEEZED LEMON JUICE

4 HARDBOILED EGGS, SHREDDED, FOR GARNISH

1 SCALLION, WHITE AND GREEN PARTS, CHOPPED, FOR GARNISH

1. Lightly grease the insert of the slow cooker with the olive oil.

2. In a medium bowl, toss together the cauliflower, bacon, pecans, garlic, salt, and pepper.

3. Transfer the mixture to the insert and sprinkle the lemon juice over the top.

4. Cover and cook on low for 6 hours.

5. Garnish with hardboiled eggs and scallion and serve.

ALLERGEN TIP: The hardboiled eggs in this recipe add protein to the finished dish, but they can be excluded if you have an allergy. Just combine this dish with a protein-rich entrée to keep your macros at the right level.

DAIRY-FREE
PALEO-FRIENDLY
QUICK PREP

KETO QUOTIENT

MACRONUTRIENTS
74% FAT
20% PROTEIN
6% CARBS

PER SERVING
CALORIES: 280
TOTAL FAT: 23G
PROTEIN: 14G
TOTAL CARBS: 9G
FIBER: 5G
NET CARBS: 4G
CHOLESTEROL: 123MG

SIMPLE SPAGHETTI SQUASH

SERVES 8 / PREP TIME: 15 MINUTES / COOK TIME: 6 HOURS ON LOW

NUT-FREE

QUICK PREP

KETO QUOTIENT

MACRONUTRIENTS
77% FAT
5% PROTEIN
8% CARBS

PER SERVING
CALORIES: 98
TOTAL FAT: 7G
PROTEIN: 1G
TOTAL CARBS: 6G
FIBER: 3G
NET CARBS: 3G
CHOLESTEROL: 15MG

Spaghetti squash shreds into charming spaghetti-like strands when it is cooked and shaved with a fork. Some people can't tell the difference between these strands and real pasta, but that usually depends on the sauce that it is mixed with. You can enjoy this dish plain or use it as a base for a more substantial dinner such as Marinara-Braised Turkey Meatballs (page 93) or Beef Goulash (page 127).

1 SMALL SPAGHETTI SQUASH, WASHED

½ CUP CHICKEN STOCK

¼ CUP BUTTER

SALT, FOR SEASONING

FRESHLY GROUND BLACK PEPPER, FOR SEASONING

1. Place the squash and chicken stock in the insert of the slow cooker. The squash should not touch the sides of the insert.

2. Cook on low for 6 hours.

3. Let the squash cool for 10 minutes and cut in half.

4. Scrape out the squash strands into a bowl with a fork. When finished, add the butter and toss to combine.

5. Season with salt and pepper and serve.

ALLERGEN TIP: Butter adds a glorious creaminess to the spaghetti squash strands and keeps them separate. You can replace the butter with 2 tablespoons of coconut oil. Pair this dish with a nice high-protein sauce or entrée to create the perfect keto combination.

KALE WITH BACON

SERVES 8 / PREP TIME: 15 MINUTES / COOK TIME: 6 HOURS ON LOW

The inspiration for this ingredient combination comes from the Southern staple of collard greens with salt pork, fatback, or ham hocks. Traditionally, the greens are slowly cooked with the meat in huge kettles for hours until they are tender. The slow cooker mimics this extended cooking time, so you will get a very similar result to the classic dish.

2 TABLESPOONS BACON FAT

2 POUNDS KALE, RINSED AND
    CHOPPED ROUGHLY

12 BACON SLICES, COOKED AND CHOPPED

2 TEASPOONS MINCED GARLIC

2 CUPS VEGETABLE BROTH

SALT, FOR SEASONING

FRESHLY GROUND BLACK PEPPER,
    FOR SEASONING

1. Generously grease the insert of the slow cooker with the bacon fat.
2. Add the kale, bacon, garlic, and broth to the insert. Gently toss to mix.
3. Cover and cook on low for 6 hours.
4. Season with salt and pepper, and serve hot.

> **VARIATION TIP:** Try other vegetables in place of the kale for interesting textures and flavors. Spinach, green beans, and bok choy all pair well with crispy bacon and garlic.

DAIRY-FREE
NUT-FREE
ALLERGEN-FREE
PALEO-FRIENDLY
QUICK PREP

KETO QUOTIENT

MACRONUTRIENTS
65% FAT
22% PROTEIN
13% CARBS

PER SERVING
CALORIES: 147
TOTAL FAT: 10G
PROTEIN: 7G
TOTAL CARBS: 7G
FIBER: 3G
NET CARBS: 4G
CHOLESTEROL: 17MG

HERBED PUMPKIN

SERVES 6 / PREP TIME: 15 MINUTES / COOK TIME: 7 TO 8 HOURS ON LOW

QUICK PREP

KETO QUOTIENT

MACRONUTRIENTS
74% FAT
10% PROTEIN
16% CARBS

PER SERVING
CALORIES: 158
TOTAL FAT: 13G
PROTEIN: 5G
TOTAL CARBS: 8G
FIBER: 3G
NET CARBS: 5G
CHOLESTEROL: 2MG

This recipe is a keto-friendly version of the mashed sweet potatoes that are popular at Thanksgiving. There is no marshmallow topping here, but you can add a generous sprinkling of chopped pecans if the giving spirit moves you. The pecans will take the macros to 82 percent fat and add 1 net carb gram to each serving.

3 TABLESPOONS EXTRA-VIRGIN OLIVE OIL, DIVIDED

1 POUND PUMPKIN, CUT INTO 1-INCH CHUNKS

½ CUP COCONUT MILK

1 TABLESPOON APPLE CIDER VINEGAR

½ TEASPOON CHOPPED THYME

1 TEASPOON CHOPPED OREGANO

¼ TEASPOON SALT

1 CUP GREEK YOGURT

1. Lightly grease the insert of the slow cooker with 1 tablespoon of the olive oil.

2. Add the remaining 2 tablespoons of the olive oil with the pumpkin, coconut milk, apple cider vinegar, thyme, oregano, and salt to the insert.

3. Cover and cook on low for 7 to 8 hours.

4. Mash the pumpkin with the yogurt using a potato masher until smooth.

5. Serve warm.

> **ALLERGEN TIP:** If you are allergic to dairy, you can mash the pumpkin with the coconut cream found at the top of canned coconut milk instead of using Greek yogurt. Simply scoop off the cream and set it aside while using the remaining coconut milk to cook the pumpkin.

GREEN BEAN CASSEROLE

SERVES 6 / PREP TIME: 15 MINUTES / COOK TIME: 6 HOURS ON LOW

Potluck dinners would not be the same without the ubiquitous condensed-mushroom-soup-and-green-bean casserole. This version does not use canned soup as a base, but it is close enough to the original to please anyone who loves its creamy taste. When served with a high-protein entrée, the macros combine perfectly for a high daily total.

¼ CUP BUTTER, DIVIDED

½ SWEET ONION, CHOPPED

1 CUP SLICED BUTTON MUSHROOMS

1 TEASPOON MINCED GARLIC

2 POUNDS GREEN BEANS, CUT INTO 2-INCH PIECES

1 CUP CHICKEN BROTH

8 OUNCES CREAM CHEESE

¼ CUP GRATED PARMESAN CHEESE

1. Lightly grease the insert of the slow cooker with 1 tablespoon of the butter.

2. In a large skillet over medium-high heat, melt the remaining butter. Add the onion, mushrooms, and garlic and sauté until the vegetables are softened, about 5 minutes.

3. Stir the green beans into the skillet and transfer the mixture to the insert.

4. In a small bowl, whisk the broth and cream cheese together until smooth.

5. Add the cheese mixture to the vegetables and stir. Top the combined mixture with the Parmesan.

6. Cover and cook on low for 6 hours.

7. Serve warm.

> **VARIATION TIP:** Try wild mushrooms instead of button mushrooms to get a different flavor. Shiitake and enoki mushrooms will add a more assertive flavor, and oyster mushrooms will create an almost-buttery texture that will be enhanced by slow cooking.

NUT-FREE

QUICK PREP

KETO QUOTIENT

MACRONUTRIENTS

72% FAT

13% PROTEIN

15% CARBS

PER SERVING

CALORIES: 274

TOTAL FAT: 22G

PROTEIN: 9G

TOTAL CARBS: 10G

FIBER: 5G

NET CARBS: 5G

CHOLESTEROL: 65MG

GOLDEN MUSHROOMS

SERVES 8 / PREP TIME: 10 MINUTES / COOK TIME: 6 HOURS ON LOW

DAIRY-FREE
NUT-FREE
ALLERGEN-FREE
PALEO-FRIENDLY
QUICK PREP

KETO QUOTIENT

MACRONUTRIENTS
80% FAT
10% PROTEIN
10% CARBS

PER SERVING
CALORIES: 58
TOTAL FAT: 5G
PROTEIN: 2G
TOTAL CARBS: 2G
FIBER: 1G
NET CARBS: 1G
CHOLESTEROL: 0MG

Mushrooms are a traditional accompaniment for grilled steak. This dish is a keto-friendly version that makes for a superlative topping. The low-carb, high-fat ratio of the dish will even out the high protein of a good steak. Choose medium-sized mushrooms, about 1½ inches in diameter so that they stay a little firm while spending hours in the slow cooker.

3 TABLESPOONS EXTRA-VIRGIN OLIVE OIL

1 POUND BUTTON MUSHROOMS, WIPED CLEAN AND HALVED

2 TEASPOONS MINCED GARLIC

¼ TEASPOON SALT

⅛ TEASPOON FRESHLY GROUND BLACK PEPPER

2 TABLESPOONS CHOPPED FRESH PARSLEY

1. Place the olive oil, mushrooms, garlic, salt, and pepper in the insert of the slow cooker and toss to coat.

2. Cover and cook on low for 6 hours.

3. Serve tossed with the parsley.

PRECOOKING TIP: Sautéing the mushrooms before adding them to the slow cooker adds an absolutely delightful color to them and can cut the cooking time by about 2 hours. Simply precook the mushrooms until they are lightly golden and fragrant.

SWEET-BRAISED RED CABBAGE

SERVES 8 / PREP TIME: 15 MINUTES / COOK TIME: 7 TO 8 HOURS ON LOW

Red cabbage becomes silky in texture and turns a glorious deep magenta color when braised. It adds spectacular color to any entrée. Do not shred the vegetable too finely because you want the individual shreds visible in the finished dish. To save time, use a food processor or mandoline to shred the cabbage quickly and uniformly.

QUICK PREP

KETO QUOTIENT

MACRONUTRIENTS
71% FAT
18% PROTEIN
11% CARBS

PER SERVING
CALORIES: 152
TOTAL FAT: 12G
PROTEIN: 7G
TOTAL CARBS: 4G
FIBER: 1G
NET CARBS: 3G
CHOLESTEROL: 13MG

1 TABLESPOON EXTRA-VIRGIN OLIVE OIL

1 SMALL RED CABBAGE, COARSELY SHREDDED (ABOUT 6 CUPS)

½ SWEET ONION, THINLY SLICED

¼ CUP APPLE CIDER VINEGAR

3 TABLESPOONS GRANULATED ERYTHRITOL

2 TEASPOONS MINCED GARLIC

½ TEASPOON GROUND NUTMEG

⅛ TEASPOON GROUND CLOVES

2 TABLESPOONS BUTTER

SALT, FOR SEASONING

FRESHLY GROUND BLACK PEPPER, FOR SEASONING

½ CUP CHOPPED WALNUTS, FOR GARNISH

½ CUP CRUMBLED BLUE CHEESE, FOR GARNISH

PINK PEPPERCORNS, FOR GARNISH (OPTIONAL)

1. Lightly grease the insert of the slow cooker with the olive oil.

2. Add the cabbage, onion, apple cider vinegar, erythritol, garlic, nutmeg, and cloves to the insert, stirring to mix well.

3. Break off little slices of butter and scatter them on top of the cabbage mixture.

4. Cover and cook on low for 7 to 8 hours.

5. Season with salt and pepper.

6. Serve topped with the walnuts, blue cheese, and peppercorns (if desired).

MAKE IT PALEO: The sweetener in this dish can be omitted and the butter replaced with coconut oil. Grass-fed butter is sometimes allowed on the Paleo diet depending on how strictly you follow the guidelines. If you eat grass-fed butter, use this kind in the recipe.

RATATOUILLE

SERVES 6 / PREP TIME: 15 MINUTES / COOK TIME: 6 HOURS ON LOW

Ratatouille is related to the French word *touiller,* meaning "to stir or toss." This peasant stew is a keto version where you will toss vegetables together to create a beautiful dish. Due to the number of vegetables used in this recipe, it is slightly higher in carbs than normally recommended for keto, but can be balanced out with other options throughout your day.

3 TABLESPOONS EXTRA-VIRGIN
   OLIVE OIL, DIVIDED

2 ZUCCHINIS, DICED

1 RED BELL PEPPER, DICED

1 YELLOW BELL PEPPER, DICED

1 CUP DICED PUMPKIN

½ SWEET ONION, DICED

3 TEASPOONS MINCED GARLIC

¼ TEASPOON SALT

¼ TEASPOON FRESHLY GROUND
   BLACK PEPPER

PINCH RED PEPPER FLAKES

1 (14-OUNCE) CAN DICED TOMATOES

1 CUP CRUMBLED GOAT CHEESE,
   FOR GARNISH

1. Lightly grease the insert of the slow cooker with 1 tablespoon of the olive oil.

2. Add the zucchini, red and yellow bell peppers, pumpkin, onion, garlic, salt, pepper, and red pepper flakes to the insert, and toss to combine.

3. Add the remaining 2 tablespoons of the olive oil and the tomatoes and stir.

4. Cover and cook on low for 6 hours.

5. Serve topped with the goat cheese.

> **MAKE IT PALEO:** Leave the goat cheese out of this recipe to create a Paleo-friendly version. This will reduce the fat and protein percentages, so serve it with a cut of meat or poultry that contains fat for a filling meal.

NORTH AFRICAN VEGETABLE STEW

SERVES 6 / PREP TIME: 15 MINUTES / COOK TIME: 7 TO 8 HOURS ON LOW

North African cuisine contains incredibly fragrant dishes. It is perfectly suited to slow cooking because the spices are meant to infuse the other ingredients with their flavors as well as their scents. The full-bodied flavor of this sauce is enhanced with peanut butter and rich coconut milk. While this stew will definitely satisfy the vegetarians in your life, it would also go well paired with lamb.

1 TABLESPOON EXTRA-VIRGIN OLIVE OIL

2 CUPS DICED PUMPKIN

2 CUPS CHOPPED CAULIFLOWER

1 RED BELL PEPPER, DICED

½ SWEET ONION, DICED

2 TEASPOONS MINCED GARLIC

2 CUPS COCONUT MILK

2 TABLESPOONS NATURAL PEANUT BUTTER

1 TABLESPOON GROUND CUMIN

1 TEASPOON GROUND CORIANDER

¼ CUP CHOPPED CILANTRO, FOR GARNISH

1. Lightly grease the insert of the slow cooker with the olive oil.

2. Add the pumpkin, cauliflower, bell pepper, onion, and garlic to the insert.

3. In a small bowl, whisk together the coconut milk, peanut butter, cumin, and coriander until smooth.

4. Pour the coconut milk mixture over the vegetables in the insert.

5. Cover and cook on low for 7 to 8 hours.

6. Serve topped with the cilantro.

> **MAKE IT PALEO:** Substitute another nut butter, such as almond butter or pecan butter, for the peanut butter in this sauce. The dish will still be delicious and retain a North African–inspired taste.

DAIRY-FREE
QUICK PREP

KETO QUOTIENT

MACRONUTRIENTS
76% FAT
11% PROTEIN
13% CARBS

PER SERVING
CALORIES: 415
TOTAL FAT: 35G
PROTEIN: 11G
TOTAL CARBS: 14G
FIBER: 7G
NET CARBS: 7G
CHOLESTEROL: 0MG

MIXED-VEGETABLE LASAGNA

SERVES 6 / PREP TIME: 20 MINUTES / COOK TIME: 7 TO 8 HOURS ON LOW

NUT-FREE

KETO QUOTIENT

MACRONUTRIENTS
70% FAT
24% PROTEIN
6% CARBS

PER SERVING
CALORIES: 345
TOTAL FAT: 25G
PROTEIN: 21G
TOTAL CARBS: 10G
FIBER: 3G
NET CARBS: 7G
CHOLESTEROL: 56MG

The long zucchini slices act as the noodles for this filling casserole, so try using a peeler to get a uniform width. Vegetable lasagna wouldn't be as fabulous without the kale or some other leafy green to add color and flavor. Kale is low in calories and carbs but helps provide volume to the dish. The leafy and trendy green is also very high in calcium, which helps burn fat and assists in attaining weight-loss goals.

3 TABLESPOONS EXTRA-VIRGIN OLIVE OIL, DIVIDED

1 CUP SLICED MUSHROOMS

2 CUPS SIMPLE MARINARA SAUCE (PAGE 165)

2 ZUCCHINI, THINLY SLICED LENGTHWISE

2 CUPS SHREDDED KALE

1 TABLESPOON CHOPPED BASIL

8 OUNCES RICOTTA CHEESE

8 OUNCES GOAT CHEESE

2 CUPS SHREDDED MOZZARELLA CHEESE

1. Lightly grease the insert of the slow cooker with 1 tablespoon olive oil.

2. In a large skillet over medium-high heat, heat the remaining 2 tablespoons of the olive oil. Add the mushrooms and sauté until they are softened, about 5 minutes.

3. Stir the marinara sauce into the mushrooms and stir to combine.

4. Pour about one-third of the sauce into the insert. Arrange one-third of the zucchini strips over the sauce. Top with one-third of the kale. Sprinkle half of both the ricotta and goat cheese over the kale. Repeat with the sauce, zucchini, kale, ricotta, and goat cheese to create another layer.

5. Top with the remaining zucchini strips and the sauce. Sprinkle the mozzarella cheese on top.

6. Cover and cook on low for 7 to 8 hours.

7. Serve warm.

PRECOOKING TIP: If you are in a rush to complete this pretty casserole, you can skip sautéing the mushrooms at the beginning of the process. This will not affect the texture or taste adversely; sautéing the mushrooms just adds a lovely golden color and richer flavor.

VEGETABLE VINDALOO

SERVES 6 / PREP TIME: 15 MINUTES / COOK TIME: 6 HOURS ON LOW

Vindaloo is one of the hottest variations of curry. Some make it painfully spicy. It originated from a Portuguese recipe, *carne de vinha d'alhos,* which was introduced to Indian culture in the fifteenth century by Portuguese sailors. The original dish featured vinegar, which is not an Indian ingredient, so broth, or coconut milk in this case, takes its place.

1 TABLESPOON EXTRA-VIRGIN OLIVE OIL

4 CUPS CAULIFLOWER FLORETS

1 CARROT, DICED

1 ZUCCHINI, DICED

1 RED BELL PEPPER, DICED

2 CUPS COCONUT MILK

½ SWEET ONION, CHOPPED

1 DRIED CHIPOTLE PEPPER, CHOPPED

1 TABLESPOON GRATED FRESH GINGER

2 TEASPOONS MINCED GARLIC

2 TEASPOONS GROUND CUMIN

1 TEASPOON GROUND CORIANDER

½ TEASPOON TURMERIC

¼ TEASPOON CAYENNE PEPPER

¼ TEASPOON CARDAMOM

1 CUP GREEK YOGURT, FOR GARNISH

2 TABLESPOONS CHOPPED CILANTRO, FOR GARNISH

1. Lightly grease the insert of the slow cooker with the olive oil.

2. Place the cauliflower, carrot, zucchini, and bell pepper in the insert.

3. In a small bowl, whisk together the coconut milk, onion, chipotle pepper, ginger, garlic, cumin, coriander, turmeric, cayenne pepper, and cardamom until well blended.

4. Pour the coconut milk mixture into the insert and stir to combine.

5. Cover and cook on low for 6 hours.

6. Serve each portion topped with the yogurt and cilantro.

ALLERGEN TIP: If you are lactose intolerant, you can either omit the yogurt or replace it with a coconut yogurt.

WILD MUSHROOM STROGANOFF

SERVES 6 / PREP TIME: 15 MINUTES / COOK TIME: 6 HOURS ON LOW

If you want a meal that is the equivalent of a warm blanket on a cold day, look no further than this recipe. The creamy, rich sauce, tender mushrooms, and gorgeous presentation make this a quintessential comfort food. You can serve leftovers over grilled steaks the next day.

3 TABLESPOONS EXTRA-VIRGIN
   OLIVE OIL, DIVIDED
2 TABLESPOONS BUTTER
14 OUNCES MUSHROOMS, SLICED
½ SWEET ONION, DICED
2 TEASPOONS MINCED GARLIC
2 CUPS BEEF BROTH

3 TABLESPOONS PAPRIKA
1 TABLESPOON TOMATO PASTE
½ CUP HEAVY (WHIPPING) CREAM
½ CUP SOUR CREAM
2 TABLESPOONS CHOPPED PARSLEY,
   FOR GARNISH

1. Lightly grease the insert of the slow cooker with 1 tablespoon of the olive oil.

2. In a large skillet over medium heat, heat the remaining 2 tablespoons of the olive oil and the butter. Add the mushrooms, onion, and garlic and sauté until they are softened, about 5 minutes.

3. Transfer the mushroom mixture to the insert and add the broth, paprika, and tomato paste.

4. Cover and cook on low for 6 hours.

5. Stir in the heavy cream and sour cream

6. Serve topped with the parsley.

> **VARIATION TIP:** You can increase the heat and earthy flavor in this creamy dish by using hot smoked paprika instead of the typical sweet paprika. Serve this dish over spiralized zucchini noodles for a real treat.

SUMMER VEGETABLE MÉLANGE

SERVES 6 / PREP TIME: 15 MINUTES / COOK TIME: 6 HOURS ON LOW

Summer markets burst with glorious vegetables perfect for side dishes and vegetarian main course choices. Try okra, pumpkin, broccoli, and Brussels sprouts in this colorful mixture if they are in season and you want to change up the ingredients. If you are serving this as a main dish, top it with a scoop of yogurt or sour cream.

½ CUP EXTRA-VIRGIN OLIVE OIL

¼ CUP BALSAMIC VINEGAR

1 TABLESPOON DRIED BASIL

1 TEASPOON DRIED THYME

¼ TEASPOON SALT

2 CUPS CAULIFLOWER FLORETS

2 ZUCCHINI, DICED INTO 1-INCH PIECES

1 YELLOW BELL PEPPER, CUT INTO STRIPS

1 CUP HALVED BUTTON MUSHROOMS

1. In a large bowl, whisk together the oil, vinegar, basil, thyme, and salt, until blended.

2. Add the cauliflower, zucchini, bell pepper, and mushrooms, and toss to coat.

3. Transfer the vegetables to the insert of a slow cooker.

4. Cover and cook on low for 6 hours.

5. Serve.

> **VARIATION TIP:** Balsamic vinegar is higher in carbs than other vinegars, about 2.3 grams per tablespoon. You can swap it out for apple cider vinegar or red wine vinegar, which has a less-sweet taste and 0 grams of carbs per tablespoon.

DAIRY-FREE
NUT-FREE
ALLERGEN-FREE
PALEO-FRIENDLY
QUICK PREP

KETO QUOTIENT

MACRONUTRIENTS
85% FAT
3% PROTEIN
12% CARBS

PER SERVING (1 CUP)
CALORIES: 189
TOTAL FAT: 18G
PROTEIN: 1G
TOTAL CARBS: 5G
FIBER: 1G
NET CARBS: 4G
CHOLESTEROL: 0MG

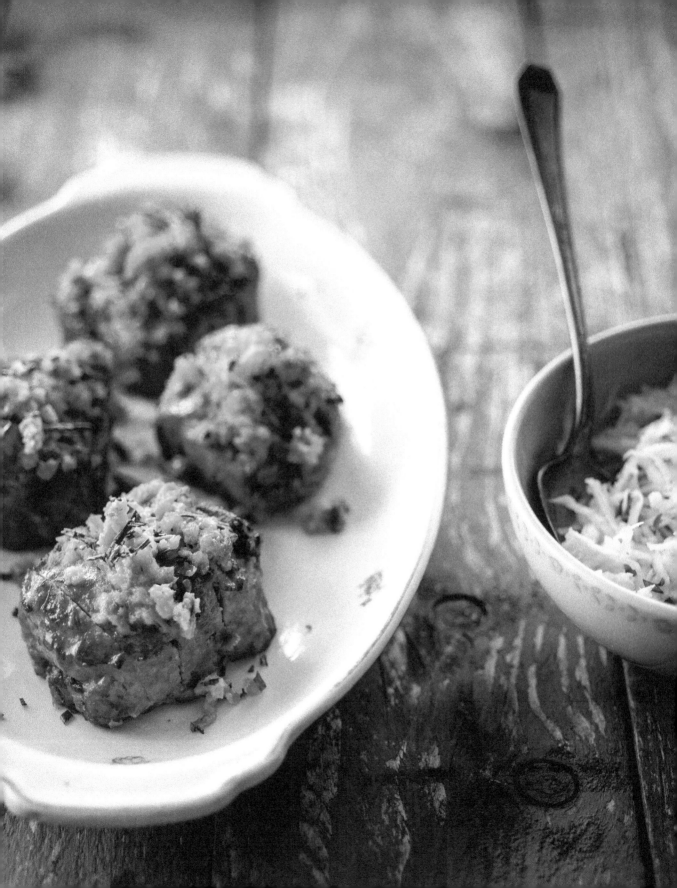

Chapter Six
POULTRY DISHES

←—a MARINARA-BRAISED TURKEY MEATBALLS, PAGE 93

BUFFALO CHICKEN

SERVES 4 / PREP TIME: 10 MINUTES / COOK TIME: 6 HOURS ON LOW

Buffalo wings are an indulgence, and creating the perfect flavor and deep-fried crispiness is almost impossible at home. But one taste of this dish will convert you to this much simpler preparation, which does not require a deep fryer and cutting whole wings into flats and drumsticks. Chicken thighs will work equally well in the sauce for the same cooking time. Just be sure to use keto-friendly hot sauce.

3 TABLESPOONS OLIVE OIL, DIVIDED

1 POUND BONELESS CHICKEN BREASTS

1 CUP HOT SAUCE

½ SWEET ONION, FINELY CHOPPED

⅓ CUP COCONUT OIL, MELTED

¼ CUP WATER

1 TEASPOON MINCED GARLIC

2 TABLESPOONS CHOPPED FRESH PARSLEY, FOR GARNISH

1. Lightly grease the insert of the slow cooker with 1 tablespoon of the olive oil.

2. In a large skillet over medium-high heat, heat the remaining 2 tablespoons of the olive oil. Add the chicken and brown for 5 minutes, turning once.

3. Transfer the chicken to the insert and arrange in one layer on the bottom.

4. In a small bowl, whisk together the hot sauce, onion, coconut oil, water, and garlic. Pour the mixture over the chicken.

5. Cover and cook on low for 6 hours.

6. Serve topped with the parsley.

VARIATION TIP: Try serving this dish topped with a scoop of blue cheese dressing to make it more decadent. It will taste like you are having baskets of chicken wings in your favorite bar. Keep in mind that if you do add blue cheese dressing, the dish will no longer be Paleo-friendly.

HUNGARIAN CHICKEN

SERVES 4 / PREP TIME: 10 MINUTES / COOK TIME: 7 TO 8 HOURS ON LOW

Sour cream is an underutilized ingredient. It can be so much more than just a topping for baked potatoes or chili. Sour cream thickens sauces, has a tangy flavor, and can provide a reasonable amount of protein and healthy fats. Make sure you purchase real sour cream rather than non-dairy versions, which are often made from hydrogenated soybean oil.

1 TABLESPOON EXTRA-VIRGIN OLIVE OIL

2 POUNDS BONELESS CHICKEN THIGHS

½ CUP CHICKEN BROTH

JUICE AND ZEST OF 1 LEMON

2 TEASPOONS MINCED GARLIC

2 TEASPOONS PAPRIKA

¼ TEASPOON SALT

1 CUP SOUR CREAM

1 TABLESPOON CHOPPED PARSLEY, FOR GARNISH

1. Lightly grease the insert of the slow cooker with the olive oil.

2. Place the chicken thighs in the insert.

3. In a small bowl, stir together the broth, lemon juice and zest, garlic, paprika, and salt. Pour the broth mixture over the chicken.

4. Cover and cook on low for 7 to 8 hours.

5. Turn off the heat and stir in the sour cream.

6. Serve topped with the parsley.

> **PRECOOKING TIP:** As with most proteins, chicken thighs can benefit from precooking in about 2 tablespoons of olive oil before adding them to the slow cooker. This step is skipped here because paprika creates a reddish hue in the sauce, so the chicken still looks delicious without searing it.

NUT-FREE
QUICK PREP

KETO QUOTIENT

MACRONUTRIENTS
73% FAT
23% PROTEIN
4% CARBS

PER SERVING
CALORIES: 404
TOTAL FAT: 32G
PROTEIN: 23G
TOTAL CARBS: 4G
FIBER: 0G
NET CARBS: 4G
CHOLESTEROL: 121MG

CREAMY LEMON CHICKEN

SERVES 6 / PREP TIME: 10 MINUTES / COOK TIME: 7 TO 8 HOURS ON LOW

NUT-FREE
QUICK PREP

KETO QUOTIENT

MACRONUTRIENTS
77% FAT
21% PROTEIN
2% CARBS

PER SERVING
CALORIES: 400
TOTAL FAT: 34G
PROTEIN: 22G
TOTAL CARBS: 2G
FIBER: 0G
NET CARBS: 2G
CHOLESTEROL: 133MG

The bright artificial-yellow sauce found in many lemon chicken dishes is very far from what you will find in this elegant meal. This lightly herbed sauce has a distinct fresh lemon flavor. The subtle color comes more from the addition of Dijon mustard, which sharpens the flavor of the other ingredients, and helps boost metabolism and immunity.

3 TABLESPOONS EXTRA-VIRGIN OLIVE OIL

2 TABLESPOONS BUTTER

1½ POUNDS BONELESS CHICKEN THIGHS

½ SWEET ONION, DICED

2 TEASPOONS MINCED GARLIC

2 TEASPOONS DRIED OREGANO

½ TEASPOON SALT

⅛ TEASPOON PEPPER, DEPENDING ON TASTE

1½ CUPS CHICKEN BROTH

JUICE AND ZEST OF 1 LEMON

1 TABLESPOON DIJON MUSTARD

1 CUP HEAVY (WHIPPING) CREAM

1. Lightly grease the insert of the slow cooker with 1 tablespoon of the olive oil.

2. In a large skillet over medium-high heat, heat the remaining 2 tablespoons of the olive oil and the butter. Add the chicken and brown for 5 minutes, turning once.

3. Transfer the chicken to the insert and add the onion, garlic, oregano, salt, and pepper.

4. In a small bowl, whisk together the broth, lemon juice and zest, and mustard. Pour the mixture over the chicken.

5. Cover and cook on low for 7 to 8 hours.

6. Remove from the heat, stir in the heavy cream, and serve.

MAKE IT PALEO: Use only extra-virgin olive oil instead of a combination of oil and butter to sear the chicken, and swap the heavy cream for coconut cream as a delicious finish for the dish.

BACON-MUSHROOM CHICKEN

SERVES 8 / PREP TIME: 15 MINUTES / COOK TIME: 7 TO 8 HOURS ON LOW

You can use bacon fat alone to brown the chicken instead of pairing it with coconut oil in this recipe. But while it would taste good, it would not give you the health benefits of coconut oil, a medium-chain triglyceride that provides quick energy and is not stored in the body as fat. It also boosts the metabolism, which in turn allows the body to burn fat faster.

3 TABLESPOONS COCONUT OIL, DIVIDED

¼ POUND BACON, DICED

2 POUNDS CHICKEN (BREASTS, THIGHS, DRUMSTICKS)

2 CUPS QUARTERED BUTTON MUSHROOMS

1 SWEET ONION, DICED

1 TABLESPOON MINCED GARLIC

½ CUP CHICKEN BROTH

2 TEASPOONS CHOPPED THYME

1 CUP COCONUT CREAM

1. Lightly grease the insert of the slow cooker with 1 tablespoon of the coconut oil.

2. In a large skillet over medium-high heat, heat the remaining 2 tablespoons of the coconut oil.

3. Add the bacon and cook until it is crispy, about 5 minutes. Using a slotted spoon, transfer the bacon to a plate and set aside.

4. Add the chicken to the skillet and brown for 5 minutes, turning once.

5. Transfer the chicken and bacon to the insert and add the mushrooms, onion, garlic, broth, and thyme.

6. Cover and cook on low for 7 to 8 hours.

7. Stir in the coconut cream and serve.

> **PRECOOKING TIP:** Cooked bacon will keep in a sealed container in the refrigerator for up to 5 days. Many keto recipes use bacon because it has a nice ratio of fat and protein, so precook a couple of packages at the beginning of the week and use them in recipes like this one.

DAIRY-FREE
ALLERGEN-FREE
PALEO-FRIENDLY
QUICK PREP

KETO QUOTIENT

MACRONUTRIENTS
71% FAT
22% PROTEIN
7% CARBS

PER SERVING
CALORIES: 406
TOTAL FAT: 34G
PROTEIN: 22G
TOTAL CARBS: 5G
FIBER: 2G
NET CARBS: 3G
CHOLESTEROL: 87MG

GARLICKY BRAISED CHICKEN THIGHS

SERVES 4 / PREP TIME: 15 MINUTES / COOK TIME: 7 TO 8 HOURS ON LOW

NUT-FREE

QUICK PREP

KETO QUOTIENT

MACRONUTRIENTS
75% FAT
20% PROTEIN
5% CARBS

PER SERVING
CALORIES: 434
TOTAL FAT: 36G
PROTEIN: 22G
TOTAL CARBS: 5G
FIBER: 1G
NET CARBS: 4G
CHOLESTEROL: 108MG

Despite the simple preparation, the flavor and delightful scent of these thighs is complex and well rounded. Topping the chicken with a generous spoon or two of creamy yogurt adds more than just a tangy taste. Yogurt is packed with gut-friendly probiotics that help reduce inflammation in the body and can reduce the amount of fat your body absorbs.

¼ CUP EXTRA-VIRGIN OLIVE OIL, DIVIDED

1½ POUNDS BONELESS CHICKEN THIGHS

1 TEASPOON PAPRIKA

SALT, FOR SEASONING

FRESHLY GROUND BLACK PEPPER,
    FOR SEASONING

1 SWEET ONION, CHOPPED

4 GARLIC CLOVES, THINLY SLICED

½ CUP CHICKEN BROTH

2 TABLESPOONS FRESHLY SQUEEZED
    LEMON JUICE

½ CUP GREEK YOGURT

1. Lightly grease the insert of the slow cooker with 1 tablespoon of the olive oil.

2. Season the thighs with paprika, salt, and pepper.

3. In a large skillet over medium-high heat, heat the remaining olive oil. Add the chicken and brown for 5 minutes, turning once.

4. Transfer the chicken to the insert and add the onion, garlic, broth, and lemon juice.

5. Cover and cook on low for 7 to 8 hours.

6. Stir in the yogurt and serve.

> **ALLERGEN TIP:** The yogurt is not crucial to the finished sauce but does add a tangy flavor and fat grams. You can leave this ingredient out if you are lactose intolerant, and the macronutrient percentage will only go down by about 2 percent fat.

COCONUT-CHICKEN CURRY

SERVES 6 / PREP TIME: 15 MINUTES / COOK TIME: 7 TO 8 HOURS ON LOW

The flavor of this complex sauce is enhanced by the addition of coconut aminos, a soy sauce substitute made from coconut sap. Coconut aminos can help regulate blood sugar and improve blood pressure with their 17 amino acids, minerals, and vitamins. The salty-sweet flavor is a perfect accompaniment for the almond butter, curry paste, and ginger.

3 TABLESPOONS EXTRA-VIRGIN OLIVE OIL, DIVIDED

1½ POUNDS BONELESS CHICKEN BREASTS

½ SWEET ONION, CHOPPED

1 CUP QUARTERED BABY BOK CHOY

1 RED BELL PEPPER, DICED

2 CUPS COCONUT MILK

2 TABLESPOONS ALMOND BUTTER

1 TABLESPOON RED THAI CURRY PASTE

1 TABLESPOON COCONUT AMINOS

2 TEASPOONS GRATED FRESH GINGER

PINCH RED PEPPER FLAKES

¼ CUP CHOPPED PEANUTS, FOR GARNISH

2 TABLESPOONS CHOPPED CILANTRO, FOR GARNISH

DAIRY-FREE
QUICK PREP

KETO QUOTIENT

MACRONUTRIENTS
70% FAT
25% PROTEIN
5% CARBS

PER SERVING
CALORIES: 543
TOTAL FAT: 42G
PROTEIN: 35G
TOTAL CARBS: 10G
FIBER: 5G
NET CARBS: 5G
CHOLESTEROL: 101MG

1. Lightly grease the insert of the slow cooker with 1 tablespoon of the olive oil.

2. In a large skillet over medium-high heat, heat the remaining 2 tablespoons of the olive oil. Add the chicken and brown for about 7 minutes.

3. Transfer the chicken to the slow cooker and add the onion, baby bok choy, and bell pepper.

4. In a medium bowl, whisk together the coconut milk, almond butter, curry paste, coconut aminos, ginger, and red pepper flakes, until well blended.

5. Pour the sauce over the chicken and vegetables, and mix to coat.

6. Cover and cook on low for 7 to 8 hours.

7. Serve topped with the peanuts and cilantro.

> **MAKE IT PALEO:** Substitute chopped peanuts for chopped almonds as a garnish. Don't worry: both add a lovely crunch and toasty flavor to the finished dish.

ONE-POT ROASTED CHICKEN DINNER

SERVES 8 / PREP TIME: 15 MINUTES / COOK TIME: 7 TO 8 HOURS ON LOW

DAIRY-FREE
NUT-FREE
ALLERGEN-FREE
PALEO-FRIENDLY
QUICK PREP

KETO QUOTIENT

MACRONUTRIENTS
73% FAT
26% PROTEIN
1% CARBS

PER SERVING
CALORIES: 427
TOTAL FAT: 34G
PROTEIN: 29G
TOTAL CARBS: 2G
FIBER: 0G
NET CARBS: 2G
CHOLESTEROL: 128MG

Roasted chicken is one of those Sunday dinner meals that requires supervision and extra work on accompaniments such as gravy or stuffing. This recipe is different. Here we are roasting a whole chicken in the slow cooker with minimal effort and preparation time, and the best part is it doesn't have to be supervised. This recipe is great if you like having cooked chicken in the refrigerator for other recipes. You can roast a whole bird at the beginning of the week and break it down as needed for later use.

¼ CUP EXTRA-VIRGIN OLIVE OIL, DIVIDED

1 (3-POUND) WHOLE CHICKEN, WASHED AND PATTED DRY

SALT, FOR SEASONING

FRESHLY GROUND BLACK PEPPER, FOR SEASONING

1 LEMON, QUARTERED

6 THYME SPRIGS

4 GARLIC CLOVES, CRUSHED

3 BAY LEAVES

1 SWEET ONION, QUARTERED

1. Lightly grease the insert of the slow cooker with 1 tablespoon of the olive oil.

2. Rub the remaining olive oil all over the chicken and season with the salt and pepper. Stuff the lemon quarters, thyme, garlic, and bay leaves into the cavity of the chicken.

3. Place the onion quarters on the bottom of the slow cooker and place the chicken on top so it does not touch the bottom of the insert.

4. Cover and cook on low for 7 to 8 hours, or until the internal temperature reaches 165°F on an instant-read thermometer.

5. Serve warm.

VARIATION TIP: Many ingredients can enhance roast chicken, which is why herbs, fruits, and vegetables are often stuffed into the cavity of this bird. You can try rosemary, limes, hot peppers, leeks, cloves, and oregano sprigs to infuse the meat with different flavors.

CHICKEN MOLE

SERVES 6 / PREP TIME: 15 MINUTES / COOK TIME: 7 TO 8 HOURS ON LOW

Mole is a Mexican classic, and its precise origins within that country are hotly disputed. Because of this, there are many different variations of this lush sauce, and it is not unusual to see in excess of 30 ingredients in each. This is a relatively simple, easy, slow cooker version.

3 TABLESPOONS EXTRA-VIRGIN OLIVE OIL OR GHEE (PAGE 158), DIVIDED

2 POUNDS BONELESS CHICKEN THIGHS AND BREASTS

SALT, FOR SEASONING

FRESHLY GROUND BLACK PEPPER, FOR SEASONING

1 SWEET ONION, CHOPPED

1 TABLESPOON MINCED GARLIC

1 (28-OUNCE) CAN DICED TOMATOES

4 DRIED CHILE PEPPERS, SOAKED IN WATER FOR 2 HOURS AND CHOPPED

3 OUNCES DARK CHOCOLATE, CHOPPED

¼ CUP NATURAL PEANUT BUTTER

1½ TEASPOONS GROUND CUMIN

¾ TEASPOON GROUND CINNAMON

½ TEASPOON CHILI POWDER

½ CUP COCONUT CREAM

2 TABLESPOONS CHOPPED CILANTRO, FOR GARNISH

QUICK PREP

KETO QUOTIENT

MACRONUTRIENTS
70% FAT
20% PROTEIN
10% CARBS

PER SERVING
CALORIES: 386
TOTAL FAT: 30G
PROTEIN: 19G
TOTAL CARBS: 11G
FIBER: 5G
NET CARBS: 6G
CHOLESTEROL: 85MG

1. Lightly grease the insert of the slow cooker with 1 tablespoon of the olive oil.

2. In a large skillet over medium-high heat, heat the remaining 2 tablespoons of the olive oil .

3. Lightly season the chicken with salt and pepper, add to the skillet, and brown for about 5 minutes, turning once.

4. Add the onion and garlic and sauté for an additional 3 minutes.

5. Transfer the chicken, onion, and garlic to the slow cooker, and stir in the tomatoes, chiles, chocolate, peanut butter, cumin, cinnamon, and chili powder.

6. Cover and cook on low for 7 to 8 hours.

7. Stir in the coconut cream, and serve hot, topped with the cilantro.

MAKE IT PALEO: Swap the peanut butter for another type of nut butter in this delectable sauce. The dark chocolate adds a glorious richness that combines well with almond butter or pecan butter.

JERK CHICKEN

SERVES 6 / PREP TIME: 15 MINUTES / COOK TIME: 7 TO 8 HOURS ON LOW

DAIRY-FREE
NUT-FREE
ALLERGEN-FREE
QUICK PREP

KETO QUOTIENT

MACRONUTRIENTS
75% FAT
22% PROTEIN
3% CARBS

PER SERVING
CALORIES: 485
TOTAL FAT: 40G
PROTEIN: 27G
TOTAL CARBS: 5G
FIBER: 1G
NET CARBS: 4G
CHOLESTEROL: 127MG

The term *jerk* refers to grilled meats flavored with a spicy-sweet mixture. While this recipe is great right out of the slow cooker, you can finish it on the grill for a more traditional flavor and presentation. If you want to cut the heat of the dish slightly, serve it with cool cucumber slices or a scoop of cold sour cream.

½ CUP EXTRA-VIRGIN OLIVE OIL, DIVIDED

2 POUNDS BONELESS CHICKEN (BREAST AND THIGHS)

1 SWEET ONION, QUARTERED

4 GARLIC CLOVES

2 SCALLIONS, WHITE AND GREEN PARTS, COARSELY CHOPPED

2 HABANERO CHILES, STEMMED AND SEEDED

2 TABLESPOONS GRANULATED ERYTHRITOL

1 TABLESPOON GRATED FRESH GINGER

2 TEASPOONS ALLSPICE

1 TEASPOON DRIED THYME

½ TEASPOON CARDAMOM

½ TEASPOON SALT

2 TABLESPOONS CHOPPED CILANTRO, FOR GARNISH

1. Lightly grease the insert of the slow cooker with 1 tablespoon of the olive oil.

2. Arrange the chicken pieces in the bottom of the insert.

3. In a blender, pulse the remaining olive oil, onion, garlic, scallions, chiles, erythritol, ginger, allspice, thyme, cardamom, and salt until a thick, uniform sauce forms.

4. Pour the sauce over the chicken, turning the pieces to coat.

5. Cover and cook on low for 7 to 8 hours.

6. Serve topped with the cilantro.

MAKE IT PALEO: This dish tastes a little more authentic with the sweetener, but the erythritol can be left out to make it conform to the Paleo diet.

CHICKEN CACCIATORE

SERVES 6 / PREP TIME: 15 MINUTES / COOK TIME: 8 HOURS ON LOW

Cacciatore means "hunter" in Italian, and modern versions of this dish feature a tomato-based sauce redolent with herbs, onion, and garlic. Traditional cacciatore does not have tomatoes, and the meat and vegetables are braised in red or white wine and stock. You can substitute rabbit for chicken if it is available.

3 TABLESPOONS EXTRA-VIRGIN
    OLIVE OIL, DIVIDED

2 POUNDS BONELESS CHICKEN THIGHS

SALT, FOR SEASONING

FRESHLY GROUND BLACK PEPPER,
    FOR SEASONING

1 (14-OUNCE) CAN STEWED TOMATOES

2 CUPS CHICKEN BROTH

1 CUP QUARTERED BUTTON MUSHROOMS

½ SWEET ONION, CHOPPED

1 TABLESPOON MINCED GARLIC

1 TABLESPOON DRIED OREGANO

1 TEASPOON DRIED BASIL

PINCH RED PEPPER FLAKES

1. Lightly grease the insert of the slow cooker with 1 tablespoon of the olive oil.

2. Lightly season the chicken thighs with salt and pepper.

3. In a large skillet over medium-high heat, heat the remaining 2 tablespoons of the olive oil. Add the chicken thighs and brown for about 8 minutes, turning once.

4. Transfer the chicken to the insert and add the tomatoes, broth, mushrooms, onion, garlic, oregano, basil, and red pepper flakes.

5. Cover and cook on low for 8 hours.

6. Serve warm.

> **VARIATION TIP:** Chicken cacciatore sounds exotic, but it is really just a humble peasant stew designed to use up ingredients. For a delectable, rich flavor, fry up 8 slices of bacon and brown the chicken thighs in the bacon fat instead of 2 tablespoons of olive oil. Add the cooked chopped bacon into the slow cooker along with the chicken thighs and other ingredients.

DAIRY-FREE
NUT-FREE
ALLERGEN-FREE
PALEO-FRIENDLY
QUICK PREP

KETO QUOTIENT

MACRONUTRIENTS
70% FAT
23% PROTEIN
7% CARBS

PER SERVING
CALORIES: 425
TOTAL FAT: 32G
PROTEIN: 27G
TOTAL CARBS: 8G
FIBER: 1G
NET CARBS: 7G
CHOLESTEROL: 128MG

EASY "ROASTED" DUCK

SERVES 8 / PREP TIME: 15 MINUTES / COOK TIME: 7 TO 8 HOURS ON LOW

DAIRY-FREE
NUT-FREE
ALLERGEN-FREE
PALEO-FRIENDLY
QUICK PREP

KETO QUOTIENT

MACRONUTRIENTS
69% FAT
29% PROTEIN
2% CARBS

PER SERVING
CALORIES: 364
TOTAL FAT: 28G
PROTEIN: 29G
TOTAL CARBS: 2G
FIBER: 1G
NET CARBS: 1G
CHOLESTEROL: 72MG

Calling this dish "roasted" might be a slightly inaccurate description, but the fragrant and incredibly juicy meat will convince you that names are not important. There is a great deal of fat in the skin of a duck, which renders out when the bird is heated. This fat will create a light golden color even in a slow cooker, especially when very little liquid is added.

3 TABLESPOONS EXTRA-VIRGIN OLIVE OIL, DIVIDED

1 (2½-POUND) WHOLE DUCK, GIBLETS REMOVED

SALT, FOR SEASONING

FRESHLY GROUND BLACK PEPPER, FOR SEASONING

4 GARLIC CLOVES, CRUSHED

6 THYME SPRIGS, CHOPPED

1 CINNAMON STICK, BROKEN INTO SEVERAL PIECES

1 SWEET ONION, COARSELY CHOPPED

¼ CUP CHICKEN BROTH

1. Lightly grease the insert of the slow cooker with 1 tablespoon of the olive oil.

2. Rub the remaining 2 tablespoons of the olive oil all over the duck and season with salt and pepper. Stuff the garlic, thyme, and cinnamon into the cavity of the duck.

3. Place the onion on the bottom of the slow cooker and place the duck on top so it does not touch the bottom of the insert, and pour in the broth.

4. Cover and cook on low for 7 to 8 hours, or until the internal temperature reaches 180°F on an instant-read thermometer.

5. Serve warm.

PRECOOKING TIP: This recipe does not call for you to do anything but rub oil on the bird. You can get ducks that are prepared to cook by the supplier, which means the skin is prerubbed, or that the bird has been boiled for several minutes so the fat renders out of the skin easily.

MARINARA-BRAISED TURKEY MEATBALLS

SERVES 6 / PREP TIME: 15 MINUTES / COOK TIME: 6 HOURS ON LOW

Meatballs are an international sensation and date back to ancient Rome, where minced meat and herbs were a common meal. Turkey is a stellar choice for meatballs because it is juicy and has a wonderful flavor. Braising the meatballs in an herbed tomato sauce adds even more taste to the dish. Serve these meatballs over spaghetti squash or zucchini noodles for a fully keto-approved meal. You can also braise the meatballs in ½ cup chicken broth if you don't want a tomato-based dish.

QUICK PREP

KETO QUOTIENT

MACRONUTRIENTS
72% FAT
25% PROTEIN
3% CARBS

PER SERVING
CALORIES: 514
TOTAL FAT: 41G
PROTEIN: 35G
TOTAL CARBS: 4G
FIBER: 1G
NET CARBS: 3G
CHOLESTEROL: 170MG

3 TABLESPOONS EXTRA-VIRGIN OLIVE OIL

1 POUND GROUND TURKEY

1 POUND BREAKFAST SAUSAGE
(PAGE 32), CRUMBLED

½ CUP ALMOND FLOUR

1 EGG

1 TABLESPOON CHOPPED BASIL

2 TEASPOONS CHOPPED OREGANO

½ TEASPOON SALT

¼ TEASPOON FRESHLY GROUND
BLACK PEPPER

2 CUPS SIMPLE MARINARA SAUCE (PAGE 165)

1 CUP SHREDDED MOZZARELLA CHEESE

1. Lightly grease the insert of the slow cooker with 1 tablespoon of the olive oil.

2. In a large bowl, mix together the turkey, sausage, almond flour, egg, basil, oregano, salt, and pepper. Roll the mixture into golf ball–sized meatballs.

3. In a large skillet over medium-high heat, heat the remaining 2 tablespoons of the olive oil. Add the meatballs and brown for 7 minutes, turning several times.

4. Transfer the meatballs to the insert and add the marinara sauce.

5. Cover and cook on low for 6 hours.

6. Serve topped with the mozzarella cheese.

> ALLERGEN TIP: The almond flour adds bulk and helps bind the other ingredients together, but it can be left out if tree nuts are a concern. Try 2 tablespoons coconut flour instead to create the proper texture.

TURKEY-PUMPKIN RAGOUT

SERVES 6 / PREP TIME: 15 MINUTES / COOK TIME: 8 HOURS ON LOW

DAIRY-FREE
ALLERGEN-FREE
PALEO-FRIENDLY
QUICK PREP

KETO QUOTIENT

MACRONUTRIENTS
70% FAT
24% PROTEIN
6% CARBS

PER SERVING
CALORIES: 418
TOTAL FAT: 34G
PROTEIN: 25G
TOTAL CARBS: 6G
FIBER: 1G
NET CARBS: 5G
CHOLESTEROL: 66MG

Ragout is the epitome of a slow-cooker dish because it is a thick stew cooked slowly over hours, which produces fork-tender meats and a savory sauce. *Ragout* comes from the French term *ragoûter*, which means "to revive the appetite." As you spoon this creamy turkey and pumpkin creation into your bowl, it certainly will!

1 TABLESPOON EXTRA-VIRGIN OLIVE OIL

1 POUND BONELESS TURKEY THIGHS, CUT INTO 1½-INCH CHUNKS

3 CUPS CUBED PUMPKIN, CUT INTO 1-INCH CHUNKS

1 RED BELL PEPPER, DICED

½ SWEET ONION, CUT IN HALF AND SLICED

1 TABLESPOON MINCED GARLIC

1½ CUPS CHICKEN BROTH

1½ CUPS COCONUT MILK

2 TEASPOONS CHOPPED FRESH THYME

½ CUP COCONUT CREAM

SALT, FOR SEASONING

FRESHLY GROUND BLACK PEPPER, FOR SEASONING

12 SLICES COOKED BACON, CHOPPED, FOR GARNISH

1. Lightly grease the insert of the slow cooker with the olive oil.

2. Add the turkey, pumpkin, red bell pepper, onion, garlic, broth, coconut milk, and thyme.

3. Cover and cook on low for 8 hours.

4. Stir in the coconut cream and season with salt and pepper.

5. Serve topped with the bacon.

PRECOOKING TIP: Browning the turkey chunks in 2 tablespoons of extra-virgin olive oil takes about 5 minutes and adds a lovely color to the meat. The added oil also bumps the keto ratio to medium.

THYME TURKEY LEGS

SERVES 6 / PREP TIME: 15 MINUTES / COOK TIME: 7 TO 8 HOURS ON LOW

Turkey legs look like something out of the medieval era, huge and comical. You will probably need to purchase two legs to get the right amount for this dish. As with most recipes, the legs will be seasoned with salt and pepper, which probably seems like an unnecessary step. Black pepper adds seasoning and seems to enhance the flavor of the meat. Black pepper can also help burn fat and can block new fat cells from forming, so don't skip the seasoning step.

3 TABLESPOONS EXTRA-VIRGIN
    OLIVE OIL, DIVIDED
2 POUNDS BONELESS TURKEY LEGS
SALT, FOR SEASONING
FRESHLY GROUND BLACK PEPPER,
    FOR SEASONING

1 TABLESPOON DRIED THYME
2 TEASPOONS POULTRY SEASONING
½ CUP CHICKEN BROTH
2 TABLESPOONS CHOPPED FRESH PARSLEY,
    FOR GARNISH

1. Lightly grease the insert of the slow cooker with 1 tablespoon of the olive oil.

2. In a large skillet over medium-high heat, heat the remaining 2 tablespoons of the olive oil.

3. Generously season the turkey with salt and pepper. Sprinkle with thyme and poultry seasoning. Add the turkey to the skillet and brown for about 7 minutes, turning once.

4. Transfer the turkey to the slow cooker and add the broth.

5. Cover and cook on low for 7 to 8 hours.

6. Serve topped with the parsley.

> **VARIATION TIP:** Herbs add complexity and fantastic flavor to meats and poultry. Turkey is a milder-tasting protein, so any type of herb or spice can enhance it. Sage, savory, marjoram, oregano, and tarragon are all inspired choices for this recipe.

DAIRY-FREE
NUT-FREE
ALLERGEN-FREE
PALEO-FRIENDLY
QUICK PREP

KETO QUOTIENT

MACRONUTRIENTS
70% FAT
29% PROTEIN
1% CARBS

PER SERVING
CALORIES: 363
TOTAL FAT: 29G
PROTEIN: 28G
TOTAL CARBS: 1G
FIBER: 0G
NET CARBS: 1G
CHOLESTEROL: 101MG

HERB-INFUSED TURKEY BREAST

SERVES 6 / PREP TIME: 25 MINUTES / COOK TIME: 7 TO 8 HOURS ON LOW

DAIRY-FREE
ALLERGEN-FREE
PALEO-FRIENDLY

KETO QUOTIENT

MACRONUTRIENTS
70% FAT
27% PROTEIN
3% CARBS

PER SERVING
CALORIES: 347
TOTAL FAT: 27G
PROTEIN: 25G
TOTAL CARBS: 5G
FIBER: 3G
NET CARBS: 2G
CHOLESTEROL: 70MG

Tender turkey breast topped with a colorful avocado salsa makes for a visually appealing feast especially when paired with Simple Spaghetti Squash (page 68) as a side. Avocado is a unique fruit, absolutely loaded with healthy fats, such as monounsaturated oleic acid, the same type found in olive oil. It also can fill you up without adding too many carbs to your daily total.

3 TABLESPOONS EXTRA-VIRGIN OLIVE OIL, DIVIDED

1½ POUNDS BONELESS TURKEY BREASTS

SALT, FOR SEASONING

FRESHLY GROUND BLACK PEPPER, FOR SEASONING

1 CUP COCONUT MILK

2 TEASPOONS MINCED GARLIC

2 TEASPOONS DRIED THYME

1 TEASPOON DRIED OREGANO

1 AVOCADO, PEELED, PITTED, AND CHOPPED

1 TOMATO, DICED

½ JALAPEÑO PEPPER, DICED

1 TABLESPOON CHOPPED CILANTRO

1. Lightly grease the insert of the slow cooker with 1 tablespoon of the olive oil.

2. In a large skillet over medium-high heat, heat the remaining 2 tablespoons of the olive oil.

3. Lightly season the turkey with salt and pepper. Add the turkey to the skillet and brown for about 7 minutes, turning once.

4. Transfer the turkey to the insert and add the coconut milk, garlic, thyme, and oregano.

5. Cover and cook on low for 7 to 8 hours.

6. In a small bowl, stir together the avocado, tomato, jalapeño pepper, and cilantro.

7. Serve the turkey topped with the avocado salsa.

PRECOOKING TIP: Although browning the turkey breast produces a lovely golden color, you do not have to sear the poultry if you remove the skin. The sauce adds moisture and flavor while cooking, and the salsa provides a splash of color to the presentation of the recipe.

HOT BUFFALO CHICKEN WINGS

SERVES 8 / PREP TIME: 10 MINUTES / COOK TIME: 6 HOURS ON LOW

Chicken wings are the perfect finger food for big family events or that lazy Sunday afternoon in front of the TV watching the game. These beauties are sticky, hot, and could be served with traditional blue cheese dressing and crudité such as carrot and celery sticks to cool your mouth.

1 (12-OUNCE) BOTTLE HOT PEPPER SAUCE

¾ CUP MELTED GRASS-FED BUTTER

1 TABLESPOON DRIED OREGANO

2 TEASPOONS GARLIC POWDER

1 TEASPOON ONION POWDER

3 POUNDS CHICKEN WING SECTIONS

1. In a large bowl, whisk together the hot sauce, butter, oregano, garlic powder, and onion powder until blended.

2. Add the chicken wings and toss to coat.

3. Pour the mixture into the insert of a slow cooker.

4. Cover and cook on low for 6 hours.

5. Serve.

> **VARIATION TIP:** If you want to create a more deep-fried look, spread the finished wings on a baking tray and bake them in the oven on 400°F for about 10 minutes, turning once.

NUT-FREE
QUICK PREP

KETO QUOTIENT

MACRONUTRIENTS
75% FAT
25% PROTEIN
0% CARBS

PER SERVING
CALORIES: 529
TOTAL FAT: 44G
PROTEIN: 31G
TOTAL CARBS: 1G
FIBER: 0G
NET CARBS: 1G
CHOLESTEROL: 175MG

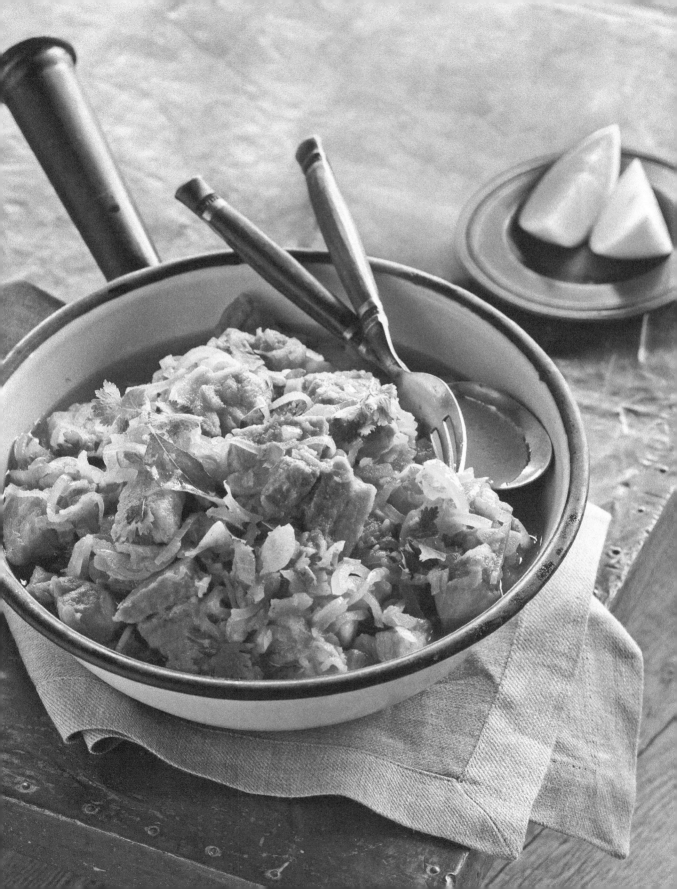

Chapter Seven
PORK & LAMB

◄─◄ CURRIED LAMB, PAGE 112

SWEET-AND-SOUR PORK CHOPS

SERVES 4 / PREP TIME: 10 MINUTES / COOK TIME: 6 HOURS ON LOW

The rose-colored sauce on these chops is probably closer to barbecue than what you would think of as sweet and sour, but the addition of coconut aminos tips the flavor into that theme. As the pork chops cook, the liquid from the broth slowly evaporates, leaving more of a glaze than a sauce on the meat. If you want the dish to have more sauce, increase the chicken broth to ¾ cup overall.

3 TABLESPOONS EXTRA-VIRGIN OLIVE OIL, DIVIDED

1 POUND BONELESS PORK CHOPS

½ CUP GRANULATED ERYTHRITOL

¼ CUP CHICKEN BROTH

¼ CUP TOMATO PASTE

2 TABLESPOONS COCONUT AMINOS

2 TABLESPOONS RED CHILI PASTE

2 TEASPOONS MINCED GARLIC

¼ TEASPOON SALT

¼ TEASPOON FRESHLY GROUND BLACK PEPPER

1. Lightly grease the insert of the slow cooker with 1 tablespoon of the olive oil.

2. In a large skillet over medium-high heat, heat the remaining 2 tablespoons of the olive oil. Add the pork chops, brown for about 5 minutes, and transfer to the insert.

3. In a medium bowl, stir together the erythritol, broth, tomato paste, coconut aminos, chili paste, garlic, salt, and pepper. Add the sauce to the chops.

4. Cover and cook on low for 6 hours.

5. Serve warm.

MAKE IT PALEO: The erythritol in the sauce obviously contributes to the sweet-and-sour theme of the dish, but you can produce a similar result with raspberry or strawberry purée. Paleo or low-carb ketchup is also quite sweet and can be used in the same amount as the sweetener.

HERB-BRAISED PORK CHOPS

SERVES 6 / PREP TIME: 15 MINUTES / COOK TIME: 7 TO 8 HOURS ON LOW

Herbs are not just culinary tools to unlocking great flavors; they also have a long history of medicinal use for many ailments. The fragrant herbs used to flavor the pork in this entrée have properties that support weight loss along with other benefits. Thyme is a powerful diuretic and oregano contains carvacrol, an active component that helps dissolve fat.

¼ CUP EXTRA-VIRGIN OLIVE OIL, DIVIDED

1½ POUNDS PORK LOIN CHOPS

SALT, FOR SEASONING

FRESHLY GROUND BLACK PEPPER, FOR SEASONING

1 CUP CHICKEN BROTH

½ SWEET ONION, CHOPPED

2 TEASPOONS MINCED GARLIC

1 TEASPOON DRIED THYME

1 TEASPOON DRIED OREGANO

1 CUP HEAVY (WHIPPING) CREAM

1 TABLESPOON CHOPPED FRESH BASIL, FOR GARNISH

1. Lightly grease the insert of the slow cooker with 1 tablespoon of the olive oil.

2. In a large skillet over medium-high heat, heat the remaining 3 tablespoons of the olive oil.

3. Lightly season the pork with salt and pepper. Add the pork to the skillet and brown for about 5 minutes. Transfer the chops to the insert.

4. In a medium bowl, stir together the broth, onion, garlic, thyme, and oregano.

5. Add the broth mixture to the chops.

6. Cover and cook on low for 7 to 8 hours.

7. Stir in the heavy cream.

8. Serve topped with the basil.

> **MAKE IT PALEO:** Use coconut milk instead of heavy cream to complete the luscious sauce. The light coconut flavor accents the pork and herbs beautifully.

NUT-FREE
QUICK PREP

KETO QUOTIENT

MACRONUTRIENTS
76% FAT
21% PROTEIN
3% CARBS

PER SERVING
CALORIES: 522
TOTAL FAT: 45G
PROTEIN: 27G
TOTAL CARBS: 2G
FIBER: 0G
NET CARBS: 2G
CHOLESTEROL: 130MG

DIJON PORK CHOPS

SERVES 4 / PREP TIME: 10 MINUTES / COOK TIME: 8 HOURS ON LOW

The pairing of maple and mustard is pure culinary magic. This sauce has a hint of heat and subtle sweetness that is further enhanced when it is blended with heavy cream and topped with fresh thyme. Since pork is a mild-flavored meat, it becomes infused with these lovely flavors as it gently braises in your slow cooker. Pork tenderloin would also work well in this recipe.

1 TABLESPOON EXTRA-VIRGIN OLIVE OIL

1 CUP CHICKEN BROTH

1 SWEET ONION, CHOPPED

¼ CUP DIJON MUSTARD

1 TEASPOON MINCED GARLIC

1 TEASPOON MAPLE EXTRACT

4 (4-OUNCE) BONELESS PORK CHOPS

1 CUP HEAVY (WHIPPING) CREAM

1 TEASPOON CHOPPED FRESH THYME, FOR GARNISH

1. Lightly grease the insert of the slow cooker with the olive oil.

2. Add the broth, onion, Dijon mustard, garlic, and maple extract to the insert, and stir to combine. Add the pork chops.

3. Cover and cook on low for 8 hours.

4. Stir in the heavy cream.

5. Serve topped with the thyme.

MAKE IT PALEO: Replace the heavy cream with coconut milk to create a lovely sauce with very little change in flavor. Dijon mustard is strong enough to mask the coconut taste, especially when it is reduced in a slow cooker.

PANCETTA-AND-BRIE-STUFFED PORK TENDERLOIN

SERVES 4 / PREP TIME: 20 MINUTES / COOK TIME: 8 HOURS ON LOW

If you have never butterflied and stuffed pork tenderloin before, you have missed out on a delectable experience. Butterflying pork is simple and just requires a sharp knife. You can stuff the pork tenderloin with other ingredients once you master the butterfly technique.

1 TABLESPOON EXTRA-VIRGIN OLIVE OIL

2 (½-POUND) PORK TENDERLOINS

4 OUNCES PANCETTA, COOKED CRISPY AND CHOPPED

4 OUNCES TRIPLE-CREAM BRIE

1 TEASPOON MINCED GARLIC

1 TEASPOON CHOPPED FRESH BASIL

⅛ TEASPOON FRESHLY GROUND BLACK PEPPER

1. Lightly grease the insert of the slow cooker with the olive oil.

2. Place the pork on a cutting board and make a lengthwise cut, holding the knife parallel to the board, through the center of the meat without cutting right through. Open the meat up like a book and cover it with plastic wrap.

3. Pound the meat with a mallet or rolling pin until each piece is about ½ inch thick. Lay the butterflied pork on a clean work surface.

4. In a small bowl, stir together the pancetta, Brie, garlic, basil, and pepper.

5. Divide the cheese mixture between the tenderloins and spread it evenly over the meat leaving about 1 inch around the edges.

6. Roll the tenderloin up and secure with toothpicks.

7. Place the pork in the insert, cover, and cook on low for 8 hours.

8. Remove the toothpicks and serve.

> **PRECOOKING TIP:** Lightly browned pork tenderloin has a delectable taste, so precooking can add to the overall appearance and taste of this dish. Simply brown the rolled pork in 1 tablespoon of olive oil for 6 minutes, turning several times. This will also increase the fat percentage of the dish.

NUT-FREE

KETO QUOTIENT

MACRONUTRIENTS
68% FAT
30% PROTEIN
2% CARBS

PER SERVING
CALORIES: 423
TOTAL FAT: 32G
PROTEIN: 34G
TOTAL CARBS: 1G
FIBER: 0G
NET CARBS: 1G
CHOLESTEROL: 132MG

LEMON PORK

SERVES 6 / PREP TIME: 15 MINUTES / COOK TIME: 7 TO 8 HOURS ON LOW

NUT-FREE
QUICK PREP

KETO QUOTIENT

MACRONUTRIENTS
65% FAT
34% PROTEIN
1% CARBS

PER SERVING
CALORIES: 448
TOTAL FAT: 31G
PROTEIN: 39G
TOTAL CARBS: 1G
FIBER: 0G
NET CARBS: 1G
CHOLESTEROL: 148MG

Pork loin roast is one of the most budget-friendly cuts of meat found in the supermarket; it is usually big enough to cut in half for two meals for a family of four. Slow cookers produce incredibly tender pork and infuse this meat with whatever flavors you add to the insert. Lemon juice and garlic create a simple but scrumptious sauce that can be spooned over a side dish as well.

3 TABLESPOONS EXTRA-VIRGIN OLIVE OIL, DIVIDED

1 TABLESPOON BUTTER

2 POUNDS PORK LOIN ROAST

½ TEASPOON SALT

¼ TEASPOON FRESHLY GROUND BLACK PEPPER

¼ CUP CHICKEN BROTH

JUICE AND ZEST OF 1 LEMON

1 TABLESPOON MINCED GARLIC

½ CUP HEAVY (WHIPPING) CREAM

1. Lightly grease the insert of the slow cooker with 1 tablespoon of the olive oil.

2. In a large skillet over medium-high heat, heat the remaining 2 tablespoons of the olive oil and the butter.

3. Lightly season the pork with salt and pepper. Add the pork to the skillet and brown the roast on all sides for about 10 minutes. Transfer it to the insert.

4. In a small bowl, stir together the broth, lemon juice and zest, and garlic.

5. Add the broth mixture to the roast.

6. Cover, and cook on low for 7 to 8 hours.

7. Stir in the heavy cream and serve.

ALLERGEN TIP: Replace the butter and heavy cream with olive oil and coconut milk, respectively, to eliminate any issues with dairy. These substitutions will also create a Paleo-friendly dish.

CRANBERRY PORK ROAST

SERVES 6 / PREP TIME: 15 MINUTES / COOK TIME: 7 TO 8 HOURS ON LOW

Although you can make this impressive-looking roast at any time of the year, the cranberries and warm spices are perfect for autumn. Cinnamon is often paired with pork, and it is a wonderful choice for anyone trying to lose or maintain weight. Cinnamon can help balance blood sugar, limit food cravings, and produce a feeling of being full.

3 TABLESPOONS EXTRA-VIRGIN OLIVE OIL, DIVIDED

2 TABLESPOONS BUTTER

2 POUNDS PORK SHOULDER ROAST

1 TEASPOON GROUND CINNAMON

¼ TEASPOON ALLSPICE

¼ TEASPOON SALT

⅛ TEASPOON FRESHLY GROUND BLACK PEPPER

½ CUP CRANBERRIES

½ CUP CHICKEN BROTH

½ CUP GRANULATED ERYTHRITOL

2 TABLESPOONS DIJON MUSTARD

JUICE AND ZEST OF ½ ORANGE

1 SCALLION, WHITE AND GREEN PARTS, CHOPPED, FOR GARNISH

1. Lightly grease the insert of the slow cooker with 1 tablespoon of the olive oil.

2. In a large skillet over medium-high heat, heat the remaining 2 tablespoons of the olive oil and the butter.

3. Lightly season the pork with cinnamon, allspice, salt, and pepper. Add the pork to the skillet and brown on all sides for about 10 minutes. Transfer to the insert.

4. In a small bowl, stir together the cranberries, broth, erythritol, mustard, and orange juice and zest, and add the mixture to the pork.

5. Cover and cook on low for 7 to 8 hours.

6. Serve topped with the scallion.

> **PRECOOKING TIP:** The tart sauce that accompanies this tender roast adds both flavor and color to the meat as it braises gently in your slow cooker. You do not have to sear the meat if you want a quicker preparation, but increase the cooking time by 1 hour if you don't.

PORK-AND-SAUERKRAUT CASSEROLE

SERVES 6 / PREP TIME: 15 MINUTES / COOK TIME: 9 TO 10 HOURS ON LOW

NUT-FREE

QUICK PREP

KETO QUOTIENT

MACRONUTRIENTS
73% FAT
22% PROTEIN
5% CARBS

PER SERVING
CALORIES: 516
TOTAL FAT: 42G
PROTEIN: 28G
TOTAL CARBS: 7G
FIBER: 4G
NET CARBS: 3G
CHOLESTEROL: 117MG

Sauerkraut is extremely healthy due to the fermentation process that produces beneficial probiotic bacteria. Pork and cabbage are often paired together because the combination produces a delightful taste and very tender meat, especially when cooked slowly with a little liquid.

3 TABLESPOONS EXTRA-VIRGIN OLIVE OIL, DIVIDED

2 TABLESPOONS BUTTER

2 POUNDS PORK SHOULDER ROAST

1 (28-OUNCE) JAR SAUERKRAUT, DRAINED

1 CUP CHICKEN BROTH

½ SWEET ONION, THINLY SLICED

¼ CUP GRANULATED ERYTHRITOL

1. Lightly grease the insert of the slow cooker with 1 tablespoon of the olive oil.

2. In a large skillet over medium-high heat, heat the remaining 2 tablespoons of the olive oil and the butter. Add the pork to the skillet and brown on all sides for about 10 minutes.

3. Transfer to the insert and add the sauerkraut, broth, onion, and erythritol.

4. Cover and cook on low for 9 to 10 hours.

5. Serve warm.

> **MAKE IT PALEO:** The butter can be replaced with olive oil, and the erythritol can be left out if you want a strict Paleo meal.

CARNITAS

SERVES 8 / PREP TIME: 15 MINUTES / COOK TIME: 9 TO 10 HOURS ON LOW

Pork is the perfect protein for dishes with lots of spices such as this succulent recipe. If you want a real treat, grind your own cumin and coriander—in a coffee grinder or with a mortar and pestle—after lightly toasting the seeds in a skillet over medium heat, swirling the skillet until the seeds are very fragrant.

3 TABLESPOONS EXTRA-VIRGIN OLIVE OIL, DIVIDED

2 POUNDS PORK SHOULDER, CUT INTO 2-INCH CUBES

2 CUPS DICED TOMATOES

2 CUPS CHICKEN BROTH

½ SWEET ONION, CHOPPED

2 FRESH CHIPOTLE PEPPERS, CHOPPED

JUICE OF 1 LIME

1 TEASPOON GROUND CORIANDER

1 TEASPOON GROUND CUMIN

½ TEASPOON SALT

1 AVOCADO, PEELED, PITTED, AND DICED, FOR GARNISH

1 CUP SOUR CREAM, FOR GARNISH

2 TABLESPOONS CHOPPED CILANTRO, FOR GARNISH

1. Lightly grease the insert of the slow cooker with 1 tablespoon of the olive oil.

2. In a large skillet over medium-high heat, heat the remaining 2 tablespoons of the olive oil.

3. Add the pork and brown on all sides for about 10 minutes.

4. Transfer to the insert and add the tomatoes, broth, onion, peppers, lime juice, coriander, cumin, and salt.

5. Cover and cook on low for 9 to 10 hours.

6. Shred the cooked pork with a fork and stir the meat into the sauce.

7. Serve topped with the avocado, sour cream, and cilantro.

> **VARIATION TIP:** Serve this flavorful meat wrapped in lettuce leaves for a handy snack or charming dinner or lunch. Try flexible leaves such as Boston lettuce or romaine with the hard center rib cut out for the best results.

NUT-FREE

QUICK PREP

KETO QUOTIENT

MACRONUTRIENTS
73% FAT
22% PROTEIN
5% CARBS

PER SERVING
CALORIES: 508
TOTAL FAT: 41G
PROTEIN: 29G
TOTAL CARBS: 7G
FIBER: 3G
NET CARBS: 4G
CHOLESTEROL: 115MG

ASIAN PORK SPARE RIBS

SERVES 4 / PREP TIME: 10 MINUTES / COOK TIME: 9 TO 10 HOURS ON LOW

Ribs are a serious undertaking for professional and amateur chefs who use rubs, smoke, sauces, and various other cooking methods to produce culinary perfection. Out of the two types of pork ribs, baby back ribs and spare ribs, the best choice for the slow cooker is spare ribs because they are fattier and get more tender the longer they cook.

1 TABLESPOON EXTRA-VIRGIN OLIVE OIL

2 POUNDS PORK SPARE RIBS

1 TABLESPOON CHINESE FIVE-SPICE POWDER

2 TEASPOONS GARLIC POWDER

½ CUP CHICKEN BROTH

3 TABLESPOONS COCONUT AMINOS

3 TABLESPOONS SESAME OIL

2 TABLESPOONS APPLE CIDER VINEGAR

1 TABLESPOON GRANULATED ERYTHRITOL

1. Lightly grease the insert of the slow cooker with the olive oil.

2. Season the ribs with the five-spice powder and garlic powder, and place upright on their ends in the insert.

3. Add the broth, coconut aminos, sesame oil, apple cider vinegar, and erythritol to the bottom of the insert, stirring to blend.

4. Cover and cook on low for 9 to 10 hours.

5. Serve warm.

MAKE IT PALEO: The rich sesame taste and saltiness of the coconut aminos can stand alone if you omit the erythritol, even though the dish will be lacking sweetness.

BACON-WRAPPED PORK LOIN

SERVES 8 / PREP TIME: 15 MINUTES / COOK TIME: 9 TO 10 HOURS ON LOW

You might decide that everything is better with bacon when you sample a slice of this seasoned bacon-wrapped pork. Depending on the shape of your pork roast, you might have to use more than eight slices of bacon to cover the surface of the meat. This addition will not change the keto macros extensively.

3 TABLESPOONS EXTRA-VIRGIN OLIVE OIL, DIVIDED

2 POUNDS PORK SHOULDER ROAST

1 TEASPOON GARLIC POWDER

1 TEASPOON ONION POWDER

8 BACON STRIPS, UNCOOKED

¼ CUP CHICKEN BROTH

2 TEASPOONS CHOPPED THYME

1 TEASPOON CHOPPED OREGANO

1. Lightly grease the insert of the slow cooker with 1 tablespoon of the olive oil.

2. Rub the pork all over with the garlic powder and onion powder.

3. In a large skillet over medium-high heat, heat the remaining 2 tablespoons of the olive oil. Add the pork to the skillet and brown on all sides for about 10 minutes. Let stand about 10 minutes to cool.

4. Wrap the pork with the bacon slices, place in the insert, and add the broth, thyme, and oregano.

5. Cover and cook on low for 9 to 10 hours.

6. Serve warm.

> **PRECOOKING TIP:** Searing the meat before wrapping it in bacon might seem like an unnecessary step because you are covering the roast anyway. Adding color and a lightly caramelized flavor to the pork creates a superior presentation and taste that you will appreciate when you slice this entrée up for family or guests.

DAIRY-FREE
NUT-FREE
ALLERGEN-FREE
PALEO-FRIENDLY
QUICK PREP

KETO QUOTIENT

MACRONUTRIENTS
73% FAT
26% PROTEIN
1% CARBS

PER SERVING
CALORIES: 493
TOTAL FAT: 40G
PROTEIN: 31G
TOTAL CARBS: 1G
FIBER: 0G
NET CARBS: 1G
CHOLESTEROL: 102MG

ALL-IN-ONE LAMB-VEGETABLE DINNER

SERVES 4 / PREP TIME: 10 MINUTES / COOK TIME: 6 HOURS ON LOW

DAIRY-FREE
NUT-FREE
ALLERGEN-FREE
PALEO-FRIENDLY
QUICK PREP

KETO QUOTIENT

MACRONUTRIENTS
77% FAT
20% PROTEIN
3% CARBS

PER SERVING
CALORIES: 431
TOTAL FAT: 37G
PROTEIN: 21G
TOTAL CARBS: 5G
FIBER: 2G
NET CARBS: 3G
CHOLESTEROL: 80MG

In this recipe, your entire dinner—entrée and side dish—will come out of the slow cooker, creating a convenient and mouthwatering meal with no stress or mess. The vegetables can be swapped for whatever you have in your refrigerator, such as cauliflower, carrots, or green beans. Add some whole crushed garlic cloves to the mix for extra flavor and nutritional benefits.

¼ CUP EXTRA-VIRGIN OLIVE OIL, DIVIDED

1 POUND BONELESS LAMB CHOPS, ABOUT ½-INCH THICK

SALT, FOR SEASONING

FRESHLY GROUND BLACK PEPPER, FOR SEASONING

½ SWEET ONION, SLICED

½ FENNEL BULB, CUT INTO 2-INCH CHUNKS

1 ZUCCHINI, CUT INTO 1-INCH CHUNKS

¼ CUP CHICKEN BROTH

2 TABLESPOONS CHOPPED FRESH BASIL, FOR GARNISH

1. Lightly grease the insert of the slow cooker with 1 tablespoon of the olive oil.

2. Season the lamb with salt and pepper.

3. In a medium bowl, toss together the onion, fennel, and zucchini with the remaining 3 tablespoons of the olive oil and then place half of the vegetables in the insert.

4. Place the lamb on top of the vegetables, cover with the remaining vegetables, and add the broth.

5. Cover and cook on low for 6 hours.

6. Serve topped with the basil.

PRECOOKING TIP: The lamb chops can be seared before placing them in the slow cooker if you want a golden finish to the meat. The lamb will be cooked through after the allotted cooking time, no matter if you precook or add the chops raw.

WILD MUSHROOM LAMB SHANKS

SERVES 6 / PREP TIME: 15 MINUTES / COOK TIME: 7 TO 8 HOURS ON LOW

Shanks are the cut of meat from below the knee and are considered to be the toughest part of the animal. Think about how active lambs are and imagine how much use these muscles get in a day. This toughness makes slow cooking the best and only option to produce a flavorsome and tender meal.

3 TABLESPOONS EXTRA-VIRGIN OLIVE OIL, DIVIDED

2 POUNDS LAMB SHANKS

½ POUND WILD MUSHROOMS, SLICED

1 LEEK, THOROUGHLY CLEANED AND CHOPPED

2 CELERY STALKS, CHOPPED

1 CARROT, DICED

1 TABLESPOON MINCED GARLIC

1 (15-OUNCE) CAN CRUSHED TOMATOES

½ CUP BEEF BROTH

2 TABLESPOONS APPLE CIDER VINEGAR

1 TEASPOON DRIED ROSEMARY

½ CUP SOUR CREAM, FOR GARNISH

1. Lightly grease the insert of the slow cooker with 1 tablespoon of the olive oil.

2. In a large skillet over medium-high heat, heat the remaining 2 tablespoons of the olive oil. Add the lamb; brown for 6 minutes, turning once; and transfer to the insert.

3. In the skillet, sauté the mushrooms, leek, celery, carrot, and garlic for 5 minutes.

4. Transfer the vegetables to the insert along with the tomatoes, broth, apple cider vinegar, and rosemary.

5. Cover and cook on low for 7 to 8 hours.

6. Serve topped with the sour cream.

> **ALLERGEN TIP:** The sour cream topping is a pretty addition, but can be left off if you want either a Paleo or dairy-free recipe. Try a scoop of either coconut cream or coconut yogurt as a suitable substitution.

NUT-FREE
QUICK PREP

KETO QUOTIENT

MACRONUTRIENTS
70% FAT
25% PROTEIN
5% CARBS

PER SERVING
CALORIES: 475
TOTAL FAT: 36G
PROTEIN: 31G
TOTAL CARBS: 11G
FIBER: 5G
NET CARBS: 6G
CHOLESTEROL: 107MG

CURRIED LAMB

SERVES 6 / PREP TIME: 15 MINUTES / COOK TIME: 7 TO 8 HOURS ON LOW

Slow cookers are ideal for curry dishes because curries benefit from long cooking times to mellow the spices and create nuances of flavor. Ginger is a common ingredient in curry blends and is used in its fresh form here. This spice can help control blood sugar, reducing glucose-level spikes after eating any carbs, and is thermogenic, meaning it helps burn fat.

3 TABLESPOONS EXTRA-VIRGIN
 OLIVE OIL, DIVIDED

1½ POUNDS LAMB SHOULDER CHOPS

SALT, FOR SEASONING

FRESHLY GROUND BLACK PEPPER,
 FOR SEASONING

3 CUPS COCONUT MILK

½ SWEET ONION, SLICED

¼ CUP CURRY POWDER

1 TABLESPOON GRATED FRESH GINGER

2 TEASPOONS MINCED GARLIC

1 CARROT, DICED

2 TABLESPOONS CHOPPED CILANTRO,
 FOR GARNISH

1. Lightly grease the insert of the slow cooker with 1 tablespoon of the olive oil.

2. In a large skillet over medium-high heat, heat the remaining 2 tablespoons of the olive oil.

3. Season the lamb with salt and pepper. Add the lamb to the skillet and brown for 6 minutes, turning once. Transfer to the insert.

4. In a medium bowl, stir together the coconut milk, onion, curry, ginger, and garlic.

5. Add the mixture to the lamb along with the carrot.

6. Cover and cook on low for 7 to 8 hours.

7. Serve topped with the cilantro.

> **PRECOOKING TIP:** This recipe has a high keto quotient, so adding the lamb chunks raw instead of searing them off is not an issue. Increase the cooking time by at least an hour to compensate for the lost time in the skillet.

ROSEMARY LAMB CHOPS

SERVES 4 / PREP TIME: 15 MINUTES / COOK TIME: 6 HOURS ON LOW

When you load this recipe into your slow cooker in the morning, the scent of rosemary and lamb will greet you at the door when you return. Rosemary is an extremely pungent herb that has a pleasing pine-like fragrance. It's used in herbal medicine to boost memory and concentration. You can use fresh rosemary in this recipe; just strip the needles off the stem and chop them finely.

3 TABLESPOONS EXTRA-VIRGIN
   OLIVE OIL, DIVIDED

1½ POUNDS LAMB SHOULDER CHOPS

SALT, FOR SEASONING

FRESHLY GROUND BLACK PEPPER,
   FOR SEASONING

½ CUP CHICKEN BROTH

1 SWEET ONION, SLICED

2 TEASPOONS MINCED GARLIC

2 TEASPOONS DRIED ROSEMARY

1 TEASPOON DRIED THYME

1. Lightly grease the insert of the slow cooker with 1 tablespoon of the olive oil.
2. In a large skillet over medium-high heat, heat the remaining 2 tablespoons of the olive oil.
3. Season the lamb with salt and pepper. Add the lamb to the skillet and brown for 6 minutes, turning once.
4. Transfer the lamb to the insert, and add the broth, onion, garlic, rosemary, and thyme.
5. Cover and cook on low for 6 hours.
6. Serve warm.

> **VARIATION TIP:** Rosemary is a classic herb for lamb, but it is not the only one that creates a perfect culinary marriage of flavors. Try chopped mint instead, either fresh or dried, for a wonderful variation on this simple recipe.

DAIRY-FREE
NUT-FREE
ALLERGEN-FREE
PALEO-FRIENDLY
QUICK PREP

KETO QUOTIENT

MACRONUTRIENTS
65% FAT
32% PROTEIN
3% CARBS

PER SERVING
CALORIES: 380
TOTAL FAT: 27G
PROTEIN: 31G
TOTAL CARBS: 3G
FIBER: 1G
NET CARBS: 2G
CHOLESTEROL: 113MG

TENDER LAMB ROAST

SERVES 6 / PREP TIME: 10 MINUTES / COOK TIME: 7 TO 8 HOURS ON LOW

NUT-FREE
QUICK PREP

KETO QUOTIENT

MACRONUTRIENTS
74% FAT
21% PROTEIN
5% CARBS

PER SERVING
CALORIES: 523
TOTAL FAT: 43G
PROTEIN: 28G
TOTAL CARBS: 6G
FIBER: 1G
NET CARBS: 5G
CHOLESTEROL: 124MG

Lamb can be an acquired taste, especially in North America, where this animal is not as popular as beef, chicken, or pork. Lamb has a gamier taste than beef that is fabulous with strong seasonings such as cumin, a spice that is used a great deal in North African and South American cuisine. It also helps out with weight-loss goals; as little as 1 teaspoon of cumin eaten daily can burn three times more body fat.

1 TABLESPOON EXTRA-VIRGIN OLIVE OIL

2 POUNDS LAMB SHOULDER ROAST

SALT, FOR SEASONING

FRESHLY GROUND BLACK PEPPER, FOR SEASONING

1 (14.5-OUNCE) CAN DICED TOMATOES

1 TABLESPOON CUMIN

2 TEASPOONS MINCED GARLIC

1 TEASPOON PAPRIKA

1 TEASPOON CHILI POWDER

1 CUP SOUR CREAM

2 TEASPOONS CHOPPED FRESH PARSLEY, FOR GARNISH

1. Lightly grease the insert of the slow cooker with the olive oil.

2. Lightly season the lamb with salt and pepper.

3. Place the lamb in the insert and add the tomatoes, cumin, garlic, paprika, and chili powder.

4. Cover and cook on low for 7 to 8 hours.

5. Stir in the sour cream.

6. Serve topped with the parsley.

> **PRECOOKING TIP:** Roasts are often precooked because slow cookers do not produce a glorious browned surface on meats. You can sear the lamb, but the flavorful cooking sauce features both paprika and chili, so color will not be an issue if you choose not to precook.

TUNISIAN LAMB RAGOUT

SERVES 6 / PREP TIME: 15 MINUTES / COOK TIME: 8 HOURS ON LOW

The spices in this fragrant meal might be unfamiliar to you although the spice mixture, *ras el hanout*, is created with many common ingredients. You will detect cinnamon, coriander, and cardamom but uncommon additions such as rose petals could be a surprise. Ras el hanout can be found in spice stores, the international section of most grocery stores, or at cooks' specialty shops.

¼ CUP EXTRA-VIRGIN OLIVE OIL

1½ POUNDS LAMB SHOULDER, CUT INTO
   1-INCH CHUNKS

1 SWEET ONION, CHOPPED

1 TABLESPOON MINCED GARLIC

4 CUPS PUMPKIN, CUT INTO 1-INCH PIECES

2 CARROTS, DICED

1 (14.5-OUNCE) CAN DICED TOMATOES

3 CUPS BEEF BROTH

2 TABLESPOONS RAS EL HANOUT

1 TEASPOON HOT CHILI POWDER

1 TEASPOON SALT

1 CUP GREEK YOGURT

1. Lightly grease the slow cooker insert with 1 tablespoon olive oil.

2. Place a large skillet over medium–high heat and add the remaining oil.

3. Brown the lamb for 6 minutes, then add the onion and garlic.

4. Sauté 3 minutes more, then transfer the lamb and vegetables to the insert.

5. Add the pumpkin, carrots, tomatoes, broth, ras el hanout, chili powder, and salt to the insert and stir to combine.

6. Cover and cook on low for 8 hours

7. Serve topped with yogurt.

> **ALLERGEN TIP:** The yogurt can be replaced with coconut cream if dairy is an issue for you. The creamy topping is there to provide a cool contrast to the spices, so make sure you thoroughly chill the coconut cream before serving.

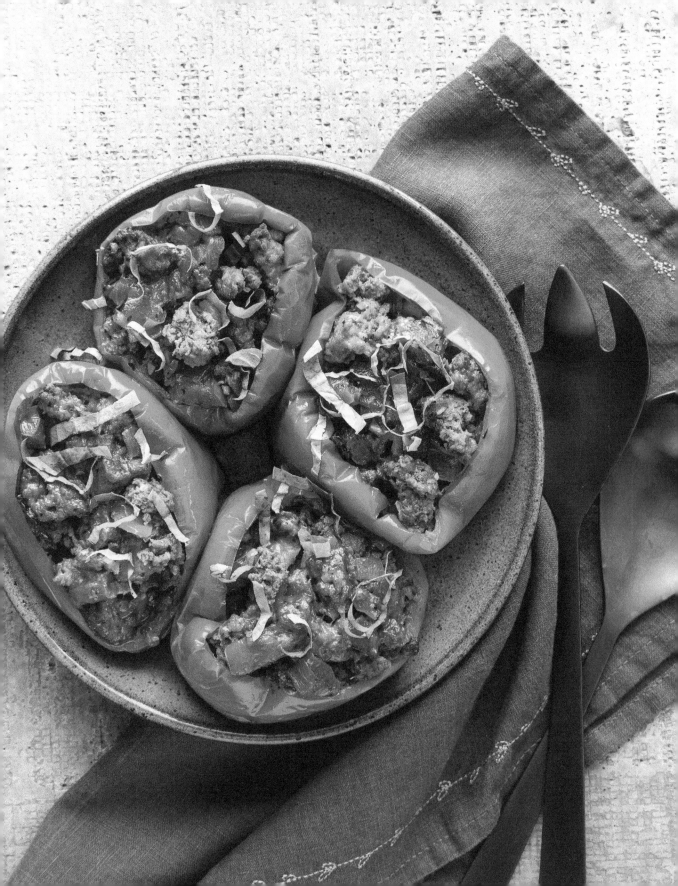

Chapter Eight
BEEF

SAVORY STUFFED PEPPERS, PAGE 132

CLASSIC SAUERBRATEN

SERVES 6 / PREP TIME: 15 MINUTES / COOK TIME: 9 TO 10 HOURS ON LOW

Brisket is a cut of beef found on the chest of the cow, and it is used for deli meats such as corned beef and pastrami. This cut is wonderful for slow cooking, especially when you ask for the "point cut" from your butcher, which has more fat. The tougher meat breaks down and gelatinizes, while the fat adds moistness and flavor.

3 TABLESPOONS EXTRA-VIRGIN
    OLIVE OIL, DIVIDED
2 POUNDS BEEF BRISKET
SALT, FOR SEASONING
FRESHLY GROUND BLACK PEPPER,
    FOR SEASONING
1 SWEET ONION, CUT INTO EIGHTHS

1 CARROT, CUT INTO CHUNKS
2 CELERY STALKS, CUT INTO CHUNKS
¾ CUP BEEF BROTH
½ CUP GERMAN-STYLE MUSTARD
¼ CUP APPLE CIDER VINEGAR
½ TEASPOON GROUND CLOVES
2 BAY LEAVES

1. Lightly grease the insert of the slow cooker with 1 tablespoon of the olive oil.

2. In a large skillet over medium-high heat, heat the remaining 2 tablespoons of the olive oil.

3. Season the beef with salt and pepper. Add the beef to the skillet and brown on all sides for 6 minutes.

4. Place the onion, carrot, and celery in the bottom of the insert and the beef on top of the vegetables.

5. In a small bowl, whisk together the broth, mustard, apple cider vinegar, and cloves, and add to the beef along with the bay leaves

6. Cover and cook on low for 9 to 10 hours.

7. Remove the bay leaves before serving.

PRECOOKING TIP: If you want to brine the brisket, you can skip the searing part of the recipe. Traditional brining does use some sugar (about 2 tablespoons) for this size roast, but it will not affect the carb count. Just soak the meat in 2 quarts water, ½ cup salt, and 2 tablespoons sugar for 7 hours in the refrigerator, and add it to the slow cooker after you remove it from the liquid and pat it dry with paper towels.

PESTO ROAST BEEF

SERVES 8 / PREP TIME: 5 MINUTES / COOK TIME: 9 TO 10 HOURS ON LOW

"Simple and quick" is how you would describe this flavorful roast. You can set the entire meal up the night before and leave the insert in the refrigerator until you are ready to cook it in the morning. Different types of pesto can be used, such as sun-dried tomato, kale, or even your own homemade version.

1 TABLESPOON EXTRA-VIRGIN OLIVE OIL

2 POUNDS BEEF CHUCK ROAST

¾ CUP PREPARED PESTO

½ CUP BEEF BROTH

1. Lightly grease the insert of the slow cooker with the olive oil.
2. Slather the pesto all over the beef. Place the beef in the insert and pour in the broth.
3. Cover and cook on low for 9 to 10 hours.
4. Serve warm.

> **PRECOOKING TIP:** If you are going to sear off this roast, do it before you spread the pesto all over the surface. You will have to wait about 10 minutes after searing because the meat will be too hot to handle right away.

QUICK PREP

KETO QUOTIENT

MACRONUTRIENTS
73% FAT
25% PROTEIN
2% CARBS

PER SERVING
CALORIES: 530
TOTAL FAT: 43G
PROTEIN: 32G
TOTAL CARBS: 2G
FIBER: 0G
NET CARBS: 2G
CHOLESTEROL: 122MG

TOMATO-BRAISED BEEF

SERVES 4 / PREP TIME: 15 MINUTES / COOK TIME: 7 TO 8 HOURS ON LOW

The reason there are so many delicious recipes combining beef and tomato is because the acid in the tomato tenderizes the meat—plus the combination tastes delicious. Braising chunks of chuck roast for hours in an herbed tomato sauce creates fork-tender meat and an incredibly rich sauce. Try serving this over zucchini noodles or Simple Spaghetti Squash (page 68).

3 TABLESPOONS EXTRA-VIRGIN OLIVE OIL, DIVIDED

1 POUND BEEF CHUCK ROAST, CUT INTO 1-INCH CUBES

SALT, FOR SEASONING

FRESHLY GROUND BLACK PEPPER, FOR SEASONING

1 (15-OUNCE) CAN DICED TOMATOES

2 TABLESPOONS TOMATO PASTE

2 TEASPOONS MINCED GARLIC

2 TEASPOONS DRIED BASIL

1 TEASPOON DRIED OREGANO

½ TEASPOON WHOLE BLACK PEPPERCORNS

1 CUP SHREDDED MOZZARELLA CHEESE, FOR GARNISH

2 TABLESPOONS CHOPPED PARSLEY, FOR GARNISH

1. Lightly grease the insert of the slow cooker with 1 tablespoon of the olive oil.

2. In a large skillet over medium-high heat, heat the remaining 2 tablespoons of the olive oil.

3. Season the beef with salt and pepper. Add the beef to the skillet and brown for 7 minutes. Transfer the beef to the insert.

4. In a medium bowl, stir together the tomatoes, tomato paste, garlic, basil, oregano, and peppercorns, and add the tomato mixture to the beef in the insert.

5. Cover and cook on low for 7 to 8 hours.

6. Serve topped with the cheese and parsley.

> **ALLERGEN TIP:** The only ingredient in this recipe that might be a problem with respect to allergies is the mozzarella cheese. If you cannot eat dairy, leave the cheesy topping off the finished dish.

BEEF AND BELL PEPPERS

SERVES 6 / PREP TIME: 15 MINUTES / COOK TIME: 9 TO 10 HOURS ON LOW

Bell peppers, with their appealing shape and wide-ranging colors, add striking appeal to any dish. This vegetable has been cultivated for hundreds of years and is valued for its sweet flavor and nutritional profile. Try to eat bell peppers soon after purchase, because the vitamin C content can drop by as much as 25 percent after 10 days in the refrigerator.

DAIRY-FREE
ALLERGEN-FREE
PALEO-FRIENDLY
QUICK PREP

KETO QUOTIENT

MACRONUTRIENTS
70% FAT
23% PROTEIN
7% CARBS

PER SERVING
CALORIES: 441
TOTAL FAT: 34G
PROTEIN: 25G
TOTAL CARBS: 11G
FIBER: 4G
NET CARBS: 7G
CHOLESTEROL: 70MG

3 TABLESPOONS EXTRA-VIRGIN OLIVE OIL, DIVIDED

1 POUND BEEF TENDERLOIN, CUT INTO 1-INCH CHUNKS

½ SWEET ONION, CHOPPED

2 TEASPOONS MINCED GARLIC

1 RED BELL PEPPER, DICED

1 YELLOW BELL PEPPER, DICED

2 CUPS COCONUT CREAM

1 CUP BEEF BROTH

3 TABLESPOONS COCONUT AMINOS

1 TABLESPOON HOT SAUCE

1 SCALLION, WHITE AND GREEN PARTS, CHOPPED, FOR GARNISH

1 TABLESPOON SESAME SEEDS, FOR GARNISH

1. Lightly grease the insert of the slow cooker with 1 tablespoon of the olive oil.

2. In a large skillet over medium-high heat, heat the remaining 2 tablespoons of the olive oil. Add the beef and brown for 6 minutes. Transfer to the insert.

3. In the skillet, sauté the onion and garlic for 3 minutes.

4. Transfer the onion and garlic to the insert along with the red pepper, yellow pepper, coconut cream, broth, coconut aminos, and hot sauce.

5. Cover and cook on low for 9 to 10 hours.

6. Serve topped with the scallion and sesame seeds.

> **VARIATION TIP:** You can enhance this simple dish by using sesame oil instead of olive oil to sear the meat. This variation will not change the macros or the keto quotient at all, and it will add an incredibly rich flavor.

SALISBURY STEAK

SERVES 6 / PREP TIME: 20 MINUTES / COOK TIME: 6 HOURS ON LOW

KETO QUOTIENT

MACRONUTRIENTS
70% FAT
26% PROTEIN
4% CARBS

PER SERVING
CALORIES: 500
TOTAL FAT: 39G
PROTEIN: 33G
TOTAL CARBS: 5G
FIBER: 2G
NET CARBS: 3G
CHOLESTEROL: 128MG

The American physician Dr. J. H. Salisbury invented the dish that bears his name over 100 years ago to support a low-carbohydrate diet for weight loss. Traditional recipes use a combination of beef and pork and do not include the almond flour that we have added here to make the recipe keto friendly. The creamy mushroom sauce and juicy patties are an enjoyable meal for the whole family.

3 TABLESPOONS EXTRA-VIRGIN OLIVE OIL, DIVIDED

1½ POUNDS GROUND BEEF

½ CUP ALMOND FLOUR

¼ CUP HEAVY (WHIPPING) CREAM

1 SCALLION, WHITE AND GREEN PARTS, CHOPPED

1 EGG

1 TEASPOON MINCED GARLIC

2 CUPS SLICED MUSHROOMS

½ SWEET ONION, CHOPPED

1½ CUPS BEEF BROTH

1 TABLESPOON DIJON MUSTARD

¾ CUP HEAVY (WHIPPING) CREAM

SALT, FOR SEASONING

FRESHLY GROUND BLACK PEPPER, FOR SEASONING

2 TABLESPOONS CHOPPED FRESH PARSLEY, FOR GARNISH

1. Lightly grease the insert of the slow cooker with 1 tablespoon of the olive oil.

2. In a medium bowl, mix together the beef, almond flour, heavy cream, scallion, egg, and garlic. Form into 6 patties about 1 inch thick.

3. In a large skillet over medium-high heat, heat the remaining 2 tablespoons of the olive oil. Pan sear the patties on both sides, about 5 minutes, and transfer the patties to the insert.

4. In the skillet, sauté the mushrooms and onion for 3 minutes.

5. Whisk in the broth and mustard and transfer the sauce to the insert.

6. Cover and cook on low for 6 hours.

7. Remove the patties to a plate and whisk the cream into the sauce.

8. Season the sauce with salt and pepper.

9. Serve the patties topped with the sauce and garnished with the parsley.

MAKE IT PALEO: Dairy cream is the traditional ingredient for Salisbury steak sauce, but it can be replaced with coconut cream to create the right texture and color. Use the same amount as the heavy cream for the best results.

GINGER BEEF

SERVES 8 / PREP TIME: 15 MINUTES / COOK TIME: 9 TO 10 HOURS ON LOW

DAIRY-FREE
NUT-FREE
ALLERGEN-FREE
QUICK PREP

KETO QUOTIENT

MACRONUTRIENTS
73% FAT
24% PROTEIN
3% CARBS

PER SERVING
CALORIES: 481
TOTAL FAT: 39G
PROTEIN: 29G
TOTAL CARBS: 4G
FIBER: 0G
NET CARBS: 4G
CHOLESTEROL: 117MG

"Ginger Beef" sounds like a dish you would order in a Chinese restaurant, but this version is more barbecue than stir-fry. Fresh ginger adds exactly the right amount of heat to the tomato-based sauce, and the apple cider vinegar brightens this delectable creation. You can serve this dish with sautéed broccoli or cauliflower for a pretty summer dinner.

¼ CUP EXTRA-VIRGIN OLIVE OIL, DIVIDED

2 POUNDS BEEF BONELESS CHUCK ROAST

½ TEASPOON SALT

½ CUP BEEF BROTH

¼ CUP PALEO OR LOW-CARB KETCHUP

2 TABLESPOONS APPLE CIDER VINEGAR

2 TABLESPOONS GRATED FRESH GINGER

1. Lightly grease the insert of the slow cooker with 1 tablespoon of the olive oil.

2. In a large skillet over medium-high heat, heat the remaining 3 tablespoons of the olive oil.

3. Season the beef with salt. Add the beef to the skillet and brown for 6 minutes. Transfer the beef to the insert.

4. In a small bowl, stir together the broth, ketchup, apple cider vinegar, and ginger. Add the broth mixture to the beef.

5. Cover and cook on low for 9 to 10 hours.

6. Serve warm.

VARIATION TIP: Fresh ginger has a slightly different taste from its dried counterpart, but you can use the dried spice if fresh is not available. Use ½ to ¾ teaspoon of dried ginger (depending on taste preference) instead of 2 tablespoons of fresh ginger.

CARNE ASADA

SERVES 8 / PREP TIME: 15 MINUTES / COOK TIME: 9 TO 10 HOURS ON LOW

If you want an authentic presentation of this dish, you will need to sear the cooked beef under the broiler until it is browned and crackly. There is a small amount of cayenne in the spice mixture, but it packs a considerable heat. Cayenne can help boost metabolism and burn up to 100 calories per meal because it raises one's body temperature.

½ CUP EXTRA-VIRGIN OLIVE OIL, DIVIDED

¼ CUP LIME JUICE

2 TABLESPOONS APPLE CIDER VINEGAR

2 TEASPOONS MINCED GARLIC

1½ TEASPOONS PAPRIKA

1 TEASPOON GROUND CUMIN

1 TEASPOON CHILI POWDER

¼ TEASPOON CAYENNE PEPPER

1 SWEET ONION CUT INTO EIGHTHS

2 POUNDS BEEF RUMP ROAST

1 CUP SOUR CREAM, FOR GARNISH

1. Lightly grease the insert of the slow cooker with 1 tablespoon of the olive oil.

2. In a small bowl, whisk together the remaining olive oil, lime juice, apple cider vinegar, garlic, paprika, cumin, chili powder, and cayenne until well blended.

3. Place the onion in the bottom of the insert and the beef on top of the vegetable. Pour the sauce over the beef.

4. Cover and cook on low for 9 to 10 hours.

5. Shred the beef with a fork.

6. Serve topped with the sour cream.

> **ALLERGEN TIP:** This recipe has a nice macro ratio of fats and protein, so eliminating the sour cream as a topping will still leave this dish suitable for keto. You can use coconut cream as a substitute if you want the keto quotient to remain higher.

NUT-FREE
QUICK PREP

KETO QUOTIENT

MACRONUTRIENTS
74% FAT
23% PROTEIN
3% CARBS

PER SERVING
CALORIES: 538
TOTAL FAT: 44G
PROTEIN: 31G
TOTAL CARBS: 3G
FIBER: 1G
NET CARBS: 2G
CHOLESTEROL: 129MG

STUFFED MEATBALLS

SERVES 6 / PREP TIME: 30 MINUTES / COOK TIME: 5 TO 6 HOURS ON LOW

NUT-FREE

KETO QUOTIENT

MACRONUTRIENTS
65% FAT
31% PROTEIN
4% CARBS

PER SERVING
CALORIES: 508
TOTAL FAT: 36G
PROTEIN: 39G
TOTAL CARBS: 6G
FIBER: 2G
NET CARBS: 4G
CHOLESTEROL: 143MG

When you bite into these herbed meatballs and encounter a hidden chunk of melted mozzarella cheese, you will be pleasantly surprised. You can prepare the meatballs ahead and freeze them on a baking tray before storing them for future use. If you are using frozen meatballs, there's no need to wait. Add the desired amount to the marinara sauce in a slow cooker and cook them for 8 to 10 hours.

3 TABLESPOONS EXTRA-VIRGIN OLIVE OIL, DIVIDED

1½ POUNDS GROUND BEEF

1 EGG

¼ CUP GRATED PARMESAN CHEESE

2 TEASPOONS MINCED GARLIC

2 TEASPOONS DRIED BASIL

½ TEASPOON SALT

¼ TEASPOON FRESHLY GROUND BLACK PEPPER

6 OUNCES MOZZARELLA, CUT INTO 16 SMALL CUBES

4 CUPS SIMPLE MARINARA SAUCE (PAGE 165)

1. Lightly grease the insert of the slow cooker with 1 tablespoon of the olive oil.

2. In large bowl, combine the beef, egg, Parmesan, garlic, basil, salt, and pepper until well mixed. Shape the mixture into 16 meatballs and press a mozzarella piece into the center of each, making sure to completely enclose the cheese.

3. In a large skillet over medium-high heat, heat the remaining 2 tablespoons of the olive oil. Add the meatballs and brown all over, about 10 minutes.

4. Transfer the meatballs to the insert and add the marinara sauce.

5. Cover and cook on low for 5 to 6 hours.

6. Serve warm.

> **ALLERGEN TIP:** One tablespoon of coconut flour can be used in place of the egg to bind the other ingredients together. Perfect firm texture is important, because you don't want the meatballs falling apart and exposing the cheesy center while they cook.

BEEF GOULASH

SERVES 6 / PREP TIME: 15 MINUTES / COOK TIME: 9 TO 10 HOURS ON LOW

There are several versions of goulash, including one with ground beef and another from the Hungarian tradition that features a thinner paprika-infused broth rather than a thick sauce. The best meat to use for this recipe is a beef cut with lots of connective tissue, such as boneless chuck. Using this kind of cut reduces the need for thickeners because it is rich in gelatin, a natural thickener.

1 TABLESPOON EXTRA-VIRGIN OLIVE OIL

1½ POUNDS BEEF, CUT INTO 1-INCH PIECES

½ SWEET ONION, CHOPPED

1 CARROT, CUT INTO ½-INCH-THICK SLICES

1 RED BELL PEPPER, DICED

2 TEASPOONS MINCED GARLIC

1 CUP BEEF BROTH

¼ CUP TOMATO PASTE

1 TABLESPOON HUNGARIAN PAPRIKA

1 BAY LEAF

1 CUP SOUR CREAM

2 TABLESPOONS CHOPPED FRESH PARSLEY, FOR GARNISH

1. Lightly grease the insert of the slow cooker with the olive oil.

2. Add the beef, onion, carrot, red bell pepper, garlic, broth, tomato paste, paprika, and bay leaf to the insert.

3. Cover and cook on low for 9 to 10 hours.

4. Remove the bay leaf and stir in the sour cream.

5. Serve topped with the parsley.

> **PRECOOKING TIP:** Searing the beef cubes before slow cooking can add fat to the dish, increasing the fat percentage by about 2 percent. As with many other recipes, the use of paprika in the sauce makes browning unnecessary.

NUT-FREE
QUICK PREP

KETO QUOTIENT

MACRONUTRIENTS
70% FAT
24% PROTEIN
6% CARBS

PER SERVING
CALORIES: 548
TOTAL FAT: 42G
PROTEIN: 32G
TOTAL CARBS: 8G
FIBER: 2G
NET CARBS: 6G
CHOLESTEROL: 134 MG

BRAISED BEEF SHORT RIBS

SERVES 8 / PREP TIME: 10 MINUTES / COOK TIME: 7 TO 8 HOURS ON LOW

**DAIRY-FREE
NUT-FREE
ALLERGEN-FREE
QUICK PREP**

KETO QUOTIENT

MACRONUTRIENTS
82% FAT
16% PROTEIN
2% CARBS

PER SERVING
CALORIES: 473
TOTAL FAT: 43G
PROTEIN: 18G
TOTAL CARBS: 2G
FIBER: 0G
NET CARBS: 2G
CHOLESTEROL: 85MG

Short ribs are from the meat cut from the first five rib bones. Since they come from an active muscle, short ribs are very flavorful but tough. You can buy the English-style one-bone chunks, or flanken-style short ribs cut into strips with three bones.

1 TABLESPOON EXTRA-VIRGIN OLIVE OIL

2 POUNDS BEEF SHORT RIBS

1 SWEET ONION, SLICED

2 CUPS BEEF BROTH

2 TABLESPOONS GRANULATED ERYTHRITOL

2 TABLESPOONS BALSAMIC VINEGAR

2 TEASPOONS DRIED THYME

1 TEASPOON HOT SAUCE

1. Lightly grease the insert of the slow cooker with the olive oil.

2. Place the ribs, onion, broth, erythritol, balsamic vinegar, thyme, and hot sauce in the insert.

3. Cover and cook on low for 7 to 8 hours.

4. Serve warm.

MAKE IT PALEO: Erythritol can be replaced by about ¼ cup strawberry purée to create the desired sweetness. The carbs in this dish are low, so the added fruit will be acceptable. And be sure to choose a Paleo-friendly hot sauce such as Frank's RedHot or Tabasco Habanero Sauce.

BALSAMIC ROAST BEEF

SERVES 8 / PREP TIME: 15 MINUTES / COOK TIME: 7 TO 8 HOURS ON LOW

Balsamic vinegar is a wonderfully sweet-and-tart combination that is superlative with beef. It has been a precious ingredient for more than 1,000 years, and prices can reach $200 per ounce for the longest-aged product. True balsamic is more of a finishing condiment, and is made in only one region in Italy, and must be aged for a minimum of 12 years to receive certification. The vinegar in your local store is most likely balsamic vinegar of Modena IGP, which still tastes lovely and is actually better for this recipe because true balsamic cannot be heated.

3 TABLESPOONS OF EXTRA-VIRGIN OLIVE OIL, DIVIDED

2 POUNDS BONELESS BEEF CHUCK ROAST

1 CUP BEEF BROTH

½ CUP BALSAMIC VINEGAR

1 TABLESPOON MINCED GARLIC

1 TABLESPOON GRANULATED ERYTHRITOL

½ TEASPOON RED PEPPER FLAKES

1 TABLESPOON CHOPPED FRESH THYME

1. Lightly grease the insert of the slow cooker with 1 tablespoon of the olive oil.

2. In a large skillet over medium-high heat, heat the remaining 2 tablespoons of the olive oil. Add the beef and brown on all sides, about 7 minutes total. Transfer to the insert.

3. In a small bowl, whisk together the broth, balsamic vinegar, garlic, erythritol, red pepper flakes, and thyme until blended.

4. Pour the sauce over the beef.

5. Cover and cook on low for 7 to 8 hours.

6. Serve warm.

> **MAKE IT PALEO:** Omit the erythritol and add 2 extra tablespoons of balsamic vinegar to the cooking liquid. Balsamic vinegar has a lovely sweetness, and this change will only add 1 carb per serving.

DAIRY-FREE
NUT-FREE
ALLERGEN-FREE
QUICK PREP

KETO QUOTIENT

MACRONUTRIENTS
74% FAT
25% PROTEIN
1% CARBS

PER SERVING
CALORIES: 476
TOTAL FAT: 39G
PROTEIN: 28G
TOTAL CARBS: 1G
FIBER: 0G
NET CARBS: 1G
CHOLESTEROL: 117MG

FIERY CURRY BEEF

SERVES 6 / PREP TIME: 10 MINUTES / COOK TIME: 7 TO 8 HOURS ON LOW

**DAIRY-FREE
ALLERGEN-FREE
PALEO-FRIENDLY
QUICK PREP**

KETO QUOTIENT

MACRONUTRIENTS
75% FAT
19% PROTEIN
6% CARBS

PER SERVING
CALORIES: 504
TOTAL FAT: 42G
PROTEIN: 23G
TOTAL CARBS: 10G
FIBER: 3G
NET CARBS: 7G
CHOLESTEROL: 78MG

Curry is a staple dish in many areas of the world, including England, where this culinary sensation is found in both high-end restaurants and food carts. Curry powder is not a singular spice but rather a combination of many different spices in varying quantities. Try mixing your own curry seasoning if you are feeling adventurous, creating a mixture that suits your palate and heat tolerance.

1 TABLESPOON EXTRA-VIRGIN OLIVE OIL

1 POUND BEEF CHUCK ROAST, CUT INTO
  2-INCH PIECES

1 SWEET ONION, CHOPPED

1 RED BELL PEPPER, DICED

2 CUPS COCONUT MILK

2 TABLESPOONS HOT CURRY POWDER

1 TABLESPOON COCONUT AMINOS

2 TEASPOONS GRATED FRESH GINGER

2 TEASPOONS MINCED GARLIC

1 CUP SHREDDED BABY BOK CHOY

1. Lightly grease the insert of the slow cooker with the olive oil.

2. Add the beef, onion, and bell pepper to the insert.

3. In a medium bowl, whisk together the coconut milk, curry, coconut aminos, ginger, and garlic. Pour the sauce into the insert and stir to combine.

4. Cover and cook on low for 7 to 8 hours.

5. Stir in the bok choy and let stand 15 minutes.

6. Serve warm.

PRECOOKING TIP: Browning the beef in this recipe can cut the cooking time down by about 2 hours. This reduced cooking time will still be sufficient to mellow the spicy sauce.

DECONSTRUCTED CABBAGE ROLLS

SERVES 4 / PREP TIME: 15 MINUTES / COOK TIME: 7 TO 8 HOURS ON LOW

Cabbage rolls can be found in many countries. This recipe is inspired by the version that is traditionally served in Russia, which has minced meat and a creamy tomato sauce. The biggest difference beyond the "deconstructed" appearance is chopped cauliflower instead of rice or buckwheat. This cruciferous vegetable is extremely high in fiber and is filling. Cauliflower also contains a decent amount of protein that balances the macro percentages perfectly.

3 TABLESPOONS EXTRA-VIRGIN OLIVE OIL, DIVIDED

1 POUND GROUND BEEF

1 SWEET ONION, CHOPPED

2 CUPS FINELY CHOPPED CAULIFLOWER

2 TEASPOONS MINCED GARLIC

1 TEASPOON DRIED THYME

¼ TEASPOON SALT

¼ TEASPOON FRESHLY GROUND BLACK PEPPER

4 CUPS SHREDDED CABBAGE

2 CUPS SIMPLE MARINARA SAUCE (PAGE 165)

½ CUP CREAM CHEESE

1. Lightly grease the insert of the slow cooker with 1 tablespoon of the olive oil.

2. Press the ground beef along bottom of the insert.

3. In a medium skillet over medium-high heat, heat the remaining 2 tablespoons of the olive oil. Add the onion, cauliflower, garlic, thyme, salt, and pepper, and sauté until the onion is softened, about 3 minutes.

4. Add the cabbage and sauté for an additional 5 minutes.

5. Transfer the cabbage mixture to the insert, pour the marinara sauce over the cabbage, and top with the cream cheese.

6. Cover and cook on low for 7 to 8 hours.

7. Stir before serving.

> **PRECOOKING TIP:** The ground beef can be cooked before placing it in the bottom of the insert if you want to reduce the cooking time to 5 to 6 hours. Cooking the beef will change the texture of the finished recipe.

NUT-FREE
QUICK PREP

KETO QUOTIENT

MACRONUTRIENTS
70% FAT
25% PROTEIN
5% CARBS

PER SERVING
CALORIES: 547
TOTAL FAT: 42G
PROTEIN: 34G
TOTAL CARBS: 10G
FIBER: 4G
NET CARBS: 6G
CHOLESTEROL: 133MG

SAVORY STUFFED PEPPERS

SERVES 4 / PREP TIME: 25 MINUTES / COOK TIME: 6 HOURS ON LOW

There is something charming about stuffed vegetables, and this is an efficient method of combining ingredients into a handy, neat package. The stuffing ingredients are a guideline rather than a strict list of what you must use in the dish. Try different ground meats, chopped vegetables, nuts, and herbs to create spectacular variations. Serve this entrée with a high-fat side dish to balance the keto macros.

3 TABLESPOONS EXTRA-VIRGIN OLIVE OIL, DIVIDED

1 POUND GROUND BEEF

½ CUP FINELY CHOPPED CAULIFLOWER

1 TOMATO, DICED

½ SWEET ONION, CHOPPED

2 TEASPOONS MINCED GARLIC

2 TEASPOONS DRIED OREGANO

1 TEASPOON DRIED BASIL

4 BELL PEPPERS, TOPS CUT OFF AND SEEDED

1 CUP SHREDDED CHEDDAR CHEESE

½ CUP CHICKEN BROTH

1 TABLESPOON BASIL, SLICED INTO THIN STRIPS, FOR GARNISH

1. Lightly grease the insert of the slow cooker with 1 tablespoon of the olive oil.

2. In a large skillet over medium-high heat, heat the remaining 2 tablespoons of the olive oil. Add the beef and sauté until it is cooked through, about 10 minutes.

3. Add the cauliflower, tomato, onion, garlic, oregano, and basil. Sauté for an additional 5 minutes.

4. Spoon the meat mixture into the bell peppers and top with the cheese.

5. Place the peppers in the slow cooker and add the broth to the bottom.

6. Cover and cook on low for 6 hours.

7. Serve warm, topped with the basil.

VARIATION TIP: Other vegetables can be used as the container for this savory filling if you are not a fan of peppers. You can also hollow out zucchini or acorn squash instead. You might have to adjust the cooking time to 8 hours or more to make up for the added vegetable size.

MEDITERRANEAN MEATLOAF

SERVES 8 / PREP TIME: 15 MINUTES / COOK TIME: 7 TO 8 HOURS ON LOW

Meatloaf takes very little time to throw together and cooking it in a slow cooker makes the task even more convenient. This old-fashioned entrée is a family favorite in many homes because it is delicious both hot and cold, with many different variations of flavors and ingredients. Try the base recipe for the loaf itself and experiment with toppings such as Asian-style glazes or Golden Caramelized Onions (page 157).

3 TABLESPOONS EXTRA-VIRGIN OLIVE OIL, DIVIDED

½ SWEET ONION, CHOPPED

2 TEASPOONS MINCED GARLIC

1 POUND GROUND BEEF

1 POUND GROUND PORK

½ CUP ALMOND FLOUR

½ CUP HEAVY (WHIPPING) CREAM

2 EGGS

2 TEASPOONS DRIED OREGANO

1 TEASPOON DRIED BASIL

¼ TEASPOON SALT

¼ TEASPOON FRESHLY GROUND BLACK PEPPER

¾ CUP TOMATO PURÉE

1 CUP GOAT CHEESE

1. Lightly grease the insert of the slow cooker with 1 tablespoon of the olive oil.

2. In a medium skillet over medium-high heat, heat the remaining 2 tablespoons of the olive oil. Add the onion and garlic and sauté until the onion is softened, about 3 minutes.

3. In a large bowl mix the onion mixture, beef, pork, almond flour, heavy cream, eggs, oregano, basil, salt, and pepper until well combined.

4. Transfer the meat mixture to the insert and form into a loaf with about ½-inch gap on the sides. Spread the tomato purée on top of the meatloaf and sprinkle with goat cheese.

5. Cover and cook on low for 7 to 8 hours.

6. Serve warm.

> **PRECOOKING TIP:** You do not have to sauté the onion and garlic if you are short on time. Just make sure that they are chopped very fine so that you don't have large, hard pieces of onion in the finished loaf.

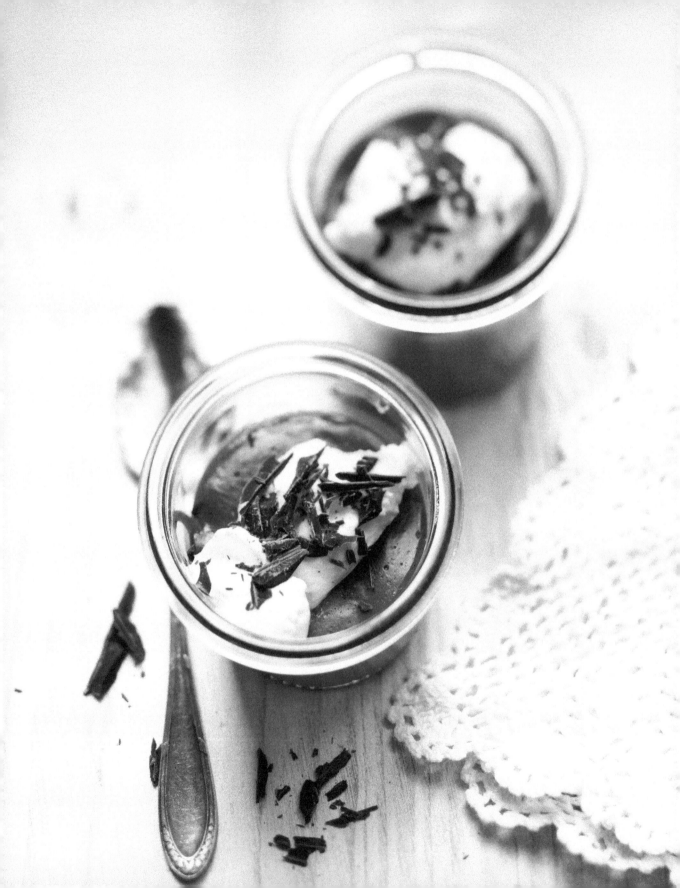

Chapter Nine

DESSERTS

← CHOCOLATE POT DE CRÈME, PAGE 136

CHOCOLATE POT DE CRÈME

SERVES 6 / PREP TIME: 10 MINUTES / COOK TIME: 3 HOURS ON LOW

NUT-FREE
QUICK PREP

KETO QUOTIENT

MACRONUTRIENTS
82% FAT
10% PROTEIN
8% CARBS

PER SERVING
CALORIES: 198
TOTAL FAT: 18G
PROTEIN: 5G
TOTAL CARBS: 4G
FIBER: 1G
NET CARBS: 3G
CHOLESTEROL: 265MG

Pot de crème is an utterly decadent chocolate pudding. Traditionally, this creation is eaten chilled so that the texture is thick and the flavor of the chocolate intense, but you can try it warm. Regardless, the scent might entice you to sample a spoonful before the baking dish makes it into the refrigerator!

6 EGG YOLKS

2 CUPS HEAVY (WHIPPING) CREAM

⅓ CUP COCOA POWDER

1 TABLESPOON PURE VANILLA EXTRACT

½ TEASPOON LIQUID STEVIA

WHIPPED COCONUT CREAM, FOR GARNISH (OPTIONAL)

SHAVED DARK CHOCOLATE, FOR GARNISH (OPTIONAL)

1. In a medium bowl, whisk together the yolks, heavy cream, cocoa powder, vanilla, and stevia.

2. Pour the mixture into a 1½-quart baking dish and place the dish in the insert of the slow cooker.

3. Pour in enough water to reach halfway up the sides of the baking dish.

4. Cover and cook on low for 3 hours.

5. Remove the baking dish from the insert and cool to room temperature on a wire rack.

6. Chill the dessert completely in the refrigerator and serve, garnished with the whipped coconut cream and shaved dark chocolate (if desired).

MAKE IT PALEO: As with many other custard desserts, dairy products such as whipping cream can be replaced with thick coconut cream. Just make sure you use a full-fat canned product rather than the watery milk found in cartons in the dairy aisle.

TEMPTING LEMON CUSTARD

SERVES 4 / PREP TIME: 10 MINUTES / COOK TIME: 3 HOURS ON LOW

Lemon is one of the most popular flavors in the world, so don't be surprised if this tangy custard disappears quickly when you serve it. The intense flavor of this dessert is enhanced by the addition of fresh lemon zest because this part of the fruit contains the essential oils. Make sure you scrub lemons very well before using them. This removes the wax applied to the skin to protect the fruit during transportation.

5 EGG YOLKS

¼ CUP FRESHLY SQUEEZED LEMON JUICE

1 TABLESPOON LEMON ZEST

1 TEASPOON PURE VANILLA EXTRACT

⅓ TEASPOON LIQUID STEVIA

2 CUPS HEAVY (WHIPPING) CREAM

1 CUP WHIPPED COCONUT CREAM
(SEE TIP ON PAGE 139)

1. In a medium bowl, whisk together the yolks, lemon juice and zest, vanilla, and liquid stevia.

2. Whisk in the heavy cream and divide the mixture between 4 (4-ounce) ramekins.

3. Place a rack at the bottom of the insert of the slow cooker and place the ramekins on it.

4. Pour in enough water to reach halfway up the sides of the ramekins.

5. Cover and cook on low for 3 hours.

6. Remove the ramekins from the insert and cool to room temperature.

7. Chill the ramekins completely in the refrigerator and serve topped with whipped coconut cream.

> **ALLERGEN TIP:** The heavy cream can be replaced by coconut cream if you have a dairy allergy. This will decrease the protein percentage in the dessert, but when combined with the other meal choices for the day, you can still end up with perfect macros.

NUT-FREE
QUICK PREP

KETO QUOTIENT

MACRONUTRIENTS
86% FAT
10% PROTEIN
4% CARBS

PER SERVING
CALORIES: 319
TOTAL FAT: 30G
PROTEIN: 7G
TOTAL CARBS: 3G
FIBER: 0G
NET CARBS: 3G
CHOLESTEROL: 365MG

PUMPKIN-GINGER PUDDING

SERVES 8 / PREP TIME: 5 MINUTES / COOK TIME: 3 TO 4 HOURS ON LOW

DAIRY-FREE
QUICK PREP

KETO QUOTIENT

MACRONUTRIENTS
78% FAT
12% PROTEIN
10% CARBS

PER SERVING
CALORIES: 217
TOTAL FAT: 19G
PROTEIN: 8G
TOTAL CARBS: 7G
FIBER: 4G
NET CARBS: 3G
CHOLESTEROL: 49MG

Puddings are a great comfort food. Think back to your childhood and how wonderful a bowl of velvety pudding made you feel. Pumpkin is a fabulous ingredient to produce those same nostalgic emotions because it contains L-tryptophan, which can create feelings of happiness. Ginger can help perk you up and reduce fatigue, so you will be happy and alert after enjoying this tasty pudding.

1 TABLESPOON COCONUT OIL

2 CUPS PUMPKIN PURÉE

1½ CUPS COCONUT MILK

2 EGGS

½ CUP ALMOND FLOUR

1 OUNCE PROTEIN POWDER

1 TABLESPOON GRATED FRESH GINGER

¾ TEASPOON LIQUID STEVIA

PINCH GROUND CLOVES

1 CUP WHIPPED COCONUT CREAM
(SEE TIP ON PAGE 139)

1. Lightly grease the insert of the slow cooker with coconut oil.

2. In a large bowl, stir together pumpkin, coconut milk, eggs, almond flour, protein powder, ginger, liquid stevia, and cloves.

3. Transfer the mixture to the insert.

4. Cover and cook on low 3 to 4 hours.

5. Serve warm with whipped coconut cream.

MAKE IT PALEO: Desserts do not have to be super sweet in order to be delightful, so taking out the liquid stevia is not a problem. Pumpkin has a lovely flavor that can be enhanced by roasting fresh pumpkin in chunks first before you mash it for this pudding.

BERRY-PUMPKIN COMPOTE

SERVES 10 / PREP TIME: 10 MINUTES / COOK TIME: 3 TO 4 HOURS ON LOW

Compote might seem like another word for jam or jelly, but there are some differences in regard to ingredients and cooking times. Compotes do not contain the pectin that causes these other recipes to firm up, and the sugar content is much lower than in jellies and jams. In this version, we have eliminated sugar completely. Compotes can be savory or sweet, and because they are slow cooked, the ingredients do not break down as much as in jams.

1 TABLESPOON COCONUT OIL

2 CUPS DICED PUMPKIN

1 CUP CRANBERRIES

1 CUP BLUEBERRIES

½ CUP GRANULATED ERYTHRITOL

JUICE AND ZEST OF 1 ORANGE

½ CUP COCONUT MILK

1 TEASPOON GROUND CINNAMON

½ TEASPOON GROUND ALLSPICE

¼ TEASPOON GROUND NUTMEG

1 CUP WHIPPED CREAM

1. Lightly grease the insert of the slow cooker with the coconut oil.

2. Place the pumpkin, cranberries, blueberries, erythritol, orange juice and zest, coconut milk, cinnamon, allspice, and nutmeg in the insert.

3. Cover and cook on low for 3 to 4 hours.

4. Let the compote cool for 1 hour and serve warm with a generous scoop of whipped cream.

> **ALLERGEN TIP:** Creating an allergen-free dessert is as easy as omitting the whipped cream topping and swapping it for whipped coconut cream. It is simple: Scoop the thick cream from the top of a can of coconut milk, and beat it until it is thick and fluffy.

SOUR-CREAM CHEESECAKE

SERVES 10 / PREP TIME: 15 MINUTES / COOK TIME: 5 TO 6 HOURS ON LOW

Cheesecake is a sublime indulgence that is the epitome of culinary achievement for chefs and home cooks alike. The quest for a perfectly luscious texture and balance of tart and sweet is a noble one. This recipe has a pureness of flavor achieved through very few ingredients.

¼ CUP BUTTER, MELTED, DIVIDED

1 CUP GROUND ALMONDS

¾ CUP PLUS 1 TABLESPOON GRANULATED ERYTHRITOL, DIVIDED

¼ TEASPOON GROUND CINNAMON

12 OUNCES CREAM CHEESE, AT ROOM TEMPERATURE

2 EGGS

2 TEASPOONS PURE VANILLA EXTRACT

1 CUP SOUR CREAM

1. Lightly grease a 7-inch springform pan with 1 tablespoon of the butter.

2. In a small bowl, stir together the almonds, 1 tablespoon of the erythritol, and cinnamon until blended.

3. Add the remaining 3 tablespoons of the butter and stir until coarse crumbs form.

4. Press the crust mixture into the springform pan along the bottom and about 2 inches up the sides.

5. In a large bowl, using a handheld mixer, beat together the cream cheese, eggs, vanilla, and remaining ¾ cup of the erythritol. Beat the sour cream into the cream-cheese mixture until smooth.

6. Spoon the batter into the springform pan and smooth out the top.

7. Place a wire rack in the insert of the slow cooker and place the springform pan on top.

8. Cover and cook on low for 5 to 6 hours, or until the cheesecake doesn't jiggle when shaken.

9. Cool completely before removing from pan.

10. Chill the cheesecake completely before serving, and store leftovers in the refrigerator.

VARIATION TIP: Try topping with fresh berries, dark chocolate, and even a drizzle of melted peanut butter to tempt your palate and delight the eyes.

PEANUT BUTTER CHEESECAKE

SERVES 10 / PREP TIME: 15 MINUTES / COOK TIME: 5 TO 6 HOURS ON LOW

Blending peanut butter and cheesecake together in one dessert leads to an exceptional creation. Cheesecake should have a velvety texture, so make sure the cream cheese and peanut butter are beaten completely smooth before adding the eggs because it is impossible to remove lumps after the batter is thinned out.

¼ CUP BUTTER, MELTED, DIVIDED

1 CUP GROUND ALMONDS

2 TABLESPOONS COCOA POWDER

1 CUP GRANULATED ERYTHRITOL, DIVIDED

12 OUNCES CREAM CHEESE, ROOM TEMPERATURE

½ CUP NATURAL PEANUT BUTTER

2 EGGS, ROOM TEMPERATURE

1 TEASPOON PURE VANILLA EXTRACT

1. Lightly grease a 7-inch springform pan with 1 tablespoon butter.

2. In a small bowl, stir together the almonds, cocoa powder, and ¼ cup erythritol until blended. Add the remaining 3 tablespoons of the butter and stir until coarse crumbs form.

3. Press the crust mixture into the springform pan along the bottom and about 2 inches up the sides.

4. In a large bowl, using a handheld mixer, beat together the cream cheese and peanut butter until smooth. Beat in the remaining ¾ cup of the erythritol, eggs, and vanilla.

5. Spoon the batter into the springform pan and smooth out the top.

6. Place a wire rack in the insert of slow cooker and place the springform pan on the wire rack.

7. Cover and cook on low for 5 to 6 hours, or until the cheesecake doesn't jiggle when shaken.

8. Cool completely before removing from pan.

9. Chill the cheesecake completely before serving, and store leftovers in the refrigerator.

> **ALLERGEN TIP:** Any other nut butter can be used instead of peanut butter in this recipe.

QUICK PREP

KETO QUOTIENT

MACRONUTRIENTS
80% FAT
14% PROTEIN
6% CARBS

PER SERVING
CALORIES: 311
TOTAL FAT: 28G
PROTEIN: 11G
TOTAL CARBS: 5G
FIBER: 2G
NET CARBS: 3G
CHOLESTEROL: 82MG

BLACKBERRY COBBLER

SERVES 10 / PREP TIME: 15 MINUTES / COOK TIME: 3 TO 4 HOURS ON LOW

QUICK PREP

KETO QUOTIENT

MACRONUTRIENTS
75% FAT
11% PROTEIN
14% CARBS

PER SERVING
CALORIES: 281
TOTAL FAT: 31G
PROTEIN: 8G
TOTAL CARBS: 10G
FIBER: 6G
NET CARBS: 4G
CHOLESTEROL: 50MG

There are many theories about how this dessert ended up with the name "cobbler"—one is that it possibly came from the spoonfuls of cakelike topping that look like cobblestones. The origin of the word also traces back to the Old English *cobeler*, meaning "wooden bowl." Whatever the history, this is a spectacularly homey dessert that is best when the berries are ripe and succulent.

FOR THE FILLING
1 TABLESPOON COCONUT OIL
6 CUPS BLACKBERRIES
½ CUP GRANULATED ERYTHRITOL
1 TEASPOON GROUND CINNAMON

FOR THE TOPPING
2 CUPS GROUND ALMONDS
½ CUP GRANULATED ERYTHRITOL
1 TABLESPOON BAKING POWDER
½ TEASPOON SALT
1 CUP HEAVY (WHIPPING) CREAM
½ CUP BUTTER, MELTED

For the filling

1. Lightly grease the insert of a 4-quart slow cooker with the coconut oil.

2. Add the blackberries, erythritol, and cinnamon to the insert. Mix to combine.

For the topping

1. In a large bowl, stir together the almonds, erythritol, baking powder, and salt. Add the heavy cream and butter and stir until a thick batter forms.

2. Drop the batter by the tablespoon on top of the blackberries.

3. Cover and cook on low for 3 to 4 hours.

4. Serve warm.

> **ALLERGEN TIP:** There is butter and heavy cream in the topping of this recipe, which is obviously an issue for people with dairy allergies. You can change the butter to coconut oil and the heavy cream to coconut milk.

BLUEBERRY CRISP

SERVES 8 / PREP TIME: 10 MINUTES / COOK TIME: 3 TO 4 HOURS ON LOW

The ground pecans add a cookielike texture to the golden, crisp topping of this dessert. Its flavor combines pleasantly with the tart, sweet berries. You can also use any other kind of berry for the filling, such as strawberries, blackberries, raspberries, or currants. If you use a slightly less sweet berry, you will probably have to add a little extra sweetener to the berry layer.

5 TABLESPOONS COCONUT OIL, MELTED, DIVIDED

4 CUPS BLUEBERRIES

¾ CUP PLUS 2 TABLESPOONS GRANULATED ERYTHRITOL

1 CUP GROUND PECANS

1 TEASPOON BAKING SODA

½ TEASPOON GROUND CINNAMON

2 TABLESPOONS COCONUT MILK

1 EGG

1. Lightly grease a 4-quart slow cooker with 1 tablespoon of the coconut oil.

2. Add the blueberries and 2 tablespoons of erythritol to the insert.

3. In a large bowl, stir together the remaining ¾ cup of the erythritol, ground pecans, baking soda, and cinnamon until well mixed.

4. Add the coconut milk, egg, and remaining coconut oil, and stir until coarse crumbs form.

5. Top the contents in the insert with the pecan mixture.

6. Cover and cook on low for 3 to 4 hours.

7. Serve warm.

> **ALLERGEN TIP:** The egg in the topping can be omitted entirely, if you don't mind a more crumbly topping on your crisp. Or you can use the flaxseed option: 1 tablespoon ground flaxseed in 3 tablespoons water chilled in the refrigerator to firm it up.

DAIRY-FREE
QUICK PREP

KETO QUOTIENT

MACRONUTRIENTS
72% FAT
14% PROTEIN
14% CARBS

PER SERVING
CALORIES: 222
TOTAL FAT: 19G
PROTEIN: 9G
TOTAL CARBS: 9G
FIBER: 4G
NET CARBS: 5G
CHOLESTEROL: 47MG

TENDER POUND CAKE

SERVES 8 / PREP TIME: 10 MINUTES / COOK TIME: 5 TO 6 HOURS ON LOW

QUICK PREP

KETO QUOTIENT

MACRONUTRIENTS
90% FAT
8% PROTEIN
2% CARBS

PER SERVING
CALORIES: 281
TOTAL FAT: 29G
PROTEIN: 5G
TOTAL CARBS: 1G
FIBER: 0G
NET CARBS: 1G
CHOLESTEROL: 163MG

This buttery dense cake originated in Northern Europe. The name comes from the earliest versions of the recipe that used 1 pound of each of the four base ingredients: flour, butter, sugar, and eggs. This recipe uses almond flour and sweetener instead of the traditional components but tastes just as delicious. This simple recipe can be enhanced with chopped nuts, different extracts such as almond or maple extract, and fresh berries baked inside.

1 TABLESPOON COCONUT OIL

2 CUPS ALMOND FLOUR

1 CUP GRANULATED ERYTHRITOL

½ TEASPOON CREAM OF TARTAR

PINCH SALT

1 CUP BUTTER, MELTED

5 EGGS

2 TEASPOONS PURE VANILLA EXTRACT

1. Lightly grease an 8-by-4-inch loaf pan with the coconut oil.
2. In a large bowl, stir together the almond flour, erythritol, cream of tartar, and salt, until well mixed.
3. In a small bowl, whisk together the butter, eggs, and vanilla.
4. Add the wet ingredients to the dry ingredients and stir to combine.
5. Transfer the batter to the loaf pan.
6. Place the loaf pan in the insert of the slow cooker.
7. Cover and cook until a toothpick inserted in the center comes out clean, about 5 to 6 hours on low.
8. Serve warm.

VARIATION TIP: Pound cake can support many different variations because the base cake has a mild taste and tender texture. You can add blueberries, a couple of tablespoons of peanut butter, mini dark chocolate chips, or lemon zest to create different spectacular cakes for any occasion.

ALMOND GOLDEN CAKE

SERVES 8 / PREP TIME: 15 MINUTES / COOK TIME: 3 HOURS ON LOW

This is a basic golden cake with a definitive almond flavor and tender, fine crumb. You can use this cake as a foundation for many dessert creations because it combines well with many flavors. If you have leftovers, don't worry, this cake freezes very well as long as it is wrapped after it is completely chilled.

½ CUP COCONUT OIL, DIVIDED

1½ CUPS ALMOND FLOUR

½ CUP COCONUT FLOUR

½ CUP GRANULATED ERYTHRITOL

2 TEASPOONS BAKING POWDER

3 EGGS

½ CUP COCONUT MILK

2 TEASPOONS PURE VANILLA EXTRACT

½ TEASPOON ALMOND EXTRACT

1. Line the insert of a 4-quart slow cooker with aluminum foil and grease the aluminum foil with 1 tablespoon of the coconut oil.

2. In a medium bowl, mix the almond flour, coconut flour, erythritol, and baking powder.

3. In a large bowl, whisk together the remaining coconut oil, eggs, coconut milk, vanilla, and almond extract.

4. Add the dry ingredients to the wet ingredients and stir until well blended.

5. Transfer the batter to the insert and use a spatula to even the top.

6. Cover and cook on low for 3 hours, or until a toothpick inserted in the center comes out clean.

7. Remove the cake from the insert and cool completely before serving.

> **VARIATION TIP:** The texture of this cake is very fine, and it can make a wonderful foundation for a pretty strawberry shortcake. Cut the finished cake into slices and top with fresh berries and a generous scoop of whipped cream.

DAIRY-FREE
QUICK PREP

KETO QUOTIENT

MACRONUTRIENTS
84% FAT
11% PROTEIN
5% CARBS

PER SERVING
CALORIES: 234
TOTAL FAT: 22G
PROTEIN: 6G
TOTAL CARBS: 3G
FIBER: 1G
NET CARBS: 2G
CHOLESTEROL: 82MG

DELECTABLE PEANUT BUTTER CUP CAKE

SERVES 8 / PREP TIME: 15 MINUTES / COOK TIME: 3 TO 4 HOURS ON LOW

QUICK PREP

KETO QUOTIENT

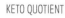

MACRONUTRIENTS
70% FAT
20% PROTEIN
10% CARBS

PER SERVING
CALORIES: 244
TOTAL FAT: 20G
PROTEIN: 11G
TOTAL CARBS: 6G
FIBER: 3G
NET CARBS: 3G
CHOLESTEROL: 10MG

Peanut butter and chocolate is a classic candy combination; it is absolutely delicious. There is no layering of flavors in this recipe so you will get an even taste of both in every delectable bite. It is an added bonus that this dessert fits the keto macros perfectly, so enjoy!

2 TABLESPOONS COCONUT OIL, DIVIDED

1 CUP ALMOND FLOUR

1 CUP GRANULATED ERYTHRITOL, DIVIDED

1 TEASPOON BAKING POWDER

¼ TEASPOON SALT

¾ CUP NATURAL PEANUT BUTTER

½ CUP HEAVY (WHIPPING) CREAM

1 TEASPOON PURE VANILLA EXTRACT

1 CUP BOILING WATER

¼ CUP COCOA POWDER

1. Lightly grease the insert of a 4-quart slow cooker with 1 tablespoon of the coconut oil.

2. In a large bowl, stir together the almond flour, ½ cup of the erythritol, baking powder, and salt.

3. In a medium bowl, whisk together the peanut butter, heavy cream, and vanilla until smooth.

4. Add the peanut butter mixture to the dry ingredients and stir to combine.

5. Transfer the batter to the insert and spread it out evenly.

6. In a small bowl, stir together the remaining ½ cup of the erythritol, boiling water, and cocoa powder.

7. Pour the chocolate mixture over the batter.

8. Cover and cook on low for 3 to 4 hours.

9. Let the cake stand for 30 minutes and serve warm.

ALLERGEN TIP: Although the classic combination that inspired the candy bar is peanut butter and chocolate, you can use almond or pecan butter instead if you are allergic to peanuts.

WARM GINGERBREAD

SERVES 8 / PREP TIME: 10 MINUTES / COOK TIME: 3 HOURS ON LOW

Gingerbread is a traditional favorite in the winter months because the spices are delicious and have been proven to support a healthy immune system. This cake has a nice light texture rather than the dense one you might be used to from your grandmother's recipe. Try making this cake topped with whipped coconut cream for a nice New Year's Day brunch, festive wedding, or birthday.

1 TABLESPOON COCONUT OIL

2 CUPS ALMOND FLOUR

¾ CUP GRANULATED ERYTHRITOL

2 TABLESPOONS COCONUT FLOUR

2 TABLESPOONS GROUND GINGER

2 TEASPOONS BAKING POWDER

2 TEASPOONS GROUND CINNAMON

½ TEASPOON GROUND NUTMEG

¼ TEASPOON GROUND CLOVES

PINCH SALT

¾ CUP HEAVY (WHIPPING) CREAM

½ CUP BUTTER, MELTED

4 EGGS

1 TEASPOON PURE VANILLA EXTRACT

1. Lightly grease the insert of the slow cooker with coconut oil.

2. In a large bowl, stir together the almond flour, erythritol, coconut flour, ginger, baking powder, cinnamon, nutmeg, cloves, and salt.

3. In a medium bowl, whisk together the heavy cream, butter, eggs, and vanilla.

4. Add the wet ingredients to the dry ingredients and stir to combine.

5. Spoon the batter into the insert.

6. Cover and cook on low for 3 hours, or until a toothpick inserted in the center comes out clean.

7. Serve warm.

> **VARIATION TIP:** The spices in this cake create a strongly flavored dessert with a bit of heat from the dried ginger. If you prefer a mellower flavor, substitute 3 tablespoons of grated fresh ginger instead.

BROWNIE CHOCOLATE CAKE

SERVES 12 / PREP TIME: 10 MINUTES / COOK TIME: 3 HOURS ON LOW

Many people feel deprived when following a specific diet plan, especially one that excludes ingredients such as sugar or flour. Fear not. This incredibly rich chocolate cake will satisfy all your dessert cravings and can be created in your slow cooker while you are using your oven for something else. If you want a more pudding-like texture in the center of the cake, cook it for only two hours instead of three.

½ CUP PLUS 1 TABLESPOON UNSALTED BUTTER, MELTED, DIVIDED

1½ CUPS ALMOND FLOUR

¾ CUP COCOA POWDER

¾ CUP GRANULATED ERYTHRITOL

1 TEASPOON BAKING POWDER

¼ TEASPOON FINE SALT

1 CUP HEAVY (WHIPPING) CREAM

3 EGGS, BEATEN

2 TEASPOONS PURE VANILLA EXTRACT

1 CUP WHIPPED CREAM

1. Generously grease the insert of the slow cooker with 1 tablespoon of the melted butter.

2. In a large bowl, stir together the almond flour, cocoa powder, erythritol, baking powder, and salt.

3. In a medium bowl, whisk together the remaining ½ cup of the melted butter, heavy cream, eggs, and vanilla until well blended.

4. Whisk the wet ingredients into the dry ingredients and spoon the batter into the insert.

5. Cover and cook on low for 3 hours, and then remove the insert from the slow cooker and let the cake sit for 1 hour.

6. Serve warm with the whipped cream.

VARIATION TIP: Brownies are the perfect base for many ingredients such as chopped pecans, dark chocolate chips, and unsweetened shredded coconut. Stir in ½ cup of any of these delectable ingredients.

LIME-RASPBERRY CUSTARD CAKE

SERVES 8 / PREP TIME: 15 MINUTES / COOK TIME: 3 HOURS ON LOW

Raspberries create jewel-like bursts of color in this lightly colored cake, in addition to creating a satisfying sweetness. Raspberries have their highest antioxidant content when they are at the peak of ripeness, so always try to purchase them in season to gain the most health benefits.

1 TEASPOON COCONUT OIL

6 EGGS, SEPARATED

2 CUPS HEAVY (WHIPPING) CREAM

¾ CUP GRANULATED ERYTHRITOL

½ CUP COCONUT FLOUR

¼ TEASPOON SALT

JUICE AND ZEST OF 2 LIMES

½ CUP RASPBERRIES

1. Lightly grease a 7-inch springform pan with the coconut oil.

2. In a large bowl, using a handheld mixer, beat the egg whites until stiff peaks form, about 5 minutes.

3. In a large bowl, whisk together the yolks, heavy cream, erythritol, coconut flour, salt, and lime juice and zest.

4. Fold the egg whites into the mixture.

5. Transfer the batter to the springform pan and sprinkle the raspberries over the top.

6. Place a wire rack in the insert of the slow cooker and place the spring-form pan on the wire rack.

7. Cover and cook on low for 3 hours, or until a toothpick inserted in the center comes out clean.

8. Remove the cover and allow the cake to cool to room temperature.

9. Place the springform pan in the refrigerator for at least 2 hours, until the cake is firm.

10. Carefully remove the sides of the springform pan. Slice and serve.

> **ALLERGEN TIP:** For those who are lactose intolerant, use coconut milk instead of heavy cream. Stir coconut cream into the coconut milk in the can to create the correct thick texture.

QUICK PREP

KETO QUOTIENT

MACRONUTRIENTS
80% FAT
15% PROTEIN
5% CARBS

PER SERVING
CALORIES: 165
TOTAL FAT: 15G
PROTEIN: 6G
TOTAL CARBS: 4G
FIBER: 1G
NET CARBS: 3G
CHOLESTEROL: 164MG

CARROT CAKE

SERVES 8 / PREP TIME: 15 MINUTES / COOK TIME: 3 HOURS ON LOW

DAIRY-FREE
QUICK PREP

KETO QUOTIENT

MACRONUTRIENTS
90% FAT
5% PROTEIN
5% CARBS

PER SERVING
CALORIES: 199
TOTAL FAT: 20G
PROTEIN: 4G
TOTAL CARBS: 4G
FIBER: 2G
NET CARBS: 2G
CHOLESTEROL: 61MG

The trick to carrot cake is finely shredded carrot rather than large pieces that do not add moisture and sweetness to every bite. Use the smallest holes on your grater to get this effect. The delicate-tasting almond flour and warm spices help create the perfect treat for a special event or birthday of a loved one. Top the cake with a generous dollop of whipped cream and a scattering of chopped pecans.

½ CUP COCONUT OIL, MELTED, DIVIDED

1 CUP GRANULATED ERYTHRITOL

2 EGGS

¼ CUP ALMOND MILK

2 TEASPOONS PURE VANILLA EXTRACT

1½ CUPS ALMOND FLOUR

1 TEASPOON BAKING POWDER

1 TEASPOON GROUND CINNAMON

½ TEASPOON BAKING SODA

½ TEASPOON GROUND GINGER

¼ TEASPOON GROUND NUTMEG

PINCH GROUND ALLSPICE

1 CUP FINELY SHREDDED CARROTS

1. Lightly grease a 7-inch springform pan with 1 tablespoon of the coconut oil.

2. In a large bowl, using a handheld mixer, beat the remaining coconut oil, erythritol, eggs, almond milk, and vanilla until blended.

3. In a medium bowl, stir together the almond flour, baking powder, cinnamon, baking soda, ginger, nutmeg, and allspice.

4. Add the dry ingredients to the wet ingredients and stir to combine.

5. Stir in the carrots until uniformly mixed.

6. Spoon the batter into the springform pan and smooth out the top.

7. Place a wire rack in the insert of the slow cooker and place the spring-form pan on the wire rack.

8. Cover and cook on low for 3 hours, or until a toothpick inserted in the center comes out clean.

9. Cool the cake and serve.

ALLERGEN TIP: If you or a loved one is allergic to tree nuts, you can make a few alterations to this recipe to create an appropriate dessert. Replace the almond flour with ½ cup coconut flour, add 2 additional eggs to the wet ingredients, and use coconut milk in the same amount as the almond milk in the recipe.

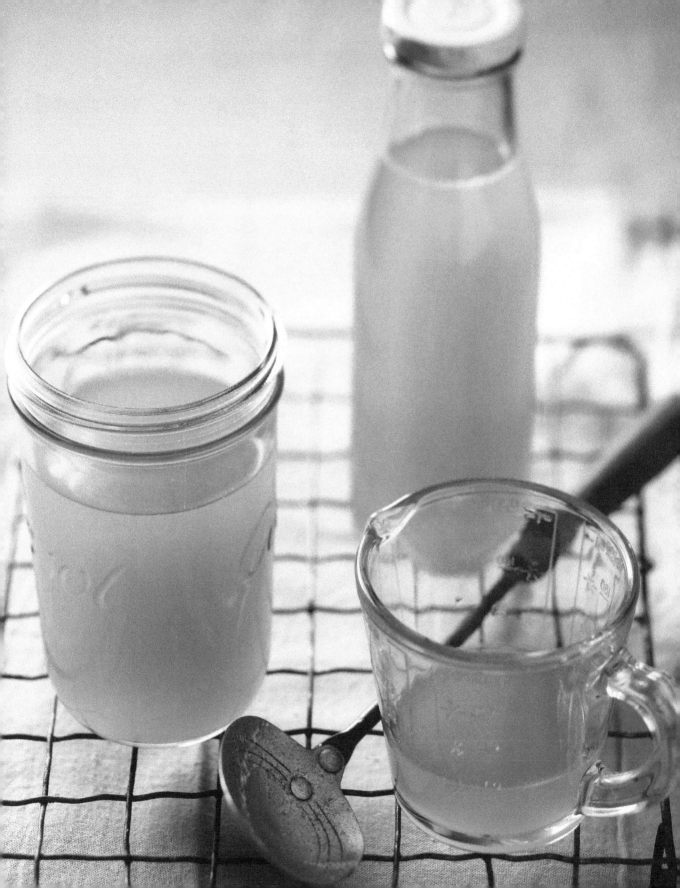

Chapter Ten

CONDIMENTS, SAUCES & BROTHS

CHICKEN BONE BROTH, PAGE 166

BACON JAM

MAKES 3 CUPS / PREP TIME: 10 MINUTES / COOK TIME: 3 TO 4 HOURS ON HIGH

Bacon jam might seem like a strange blend of ingredients unless you have ever had bacon dipped into maple syrup or dark chocolate. The sweet, tangy, and savory combination is exquisite and seems to spark every taste bud in your mouth. Try a spoonful of this delightful jam on a steak, burger, or roasted pork chop.

3 TABLESPOONS BACON FAT, MELTED AND DIVIDED

1 POUND COOKED BACON, CHOPPED INTO ½-INCH PIECES

1 SWEET ONION, DICED

½ CUP APPLE CIDER VINEGAR

¼ CUP GRANULATED ERYTHRITOL

1 TABLESPOON MINCED GARLIC

1 CUP BREWED DECAFFEINATED COFFEE

1. Lightly grease the insert of the slow cooker with 1 tablespoon of the bacon fat.

2. Add the remaining 2 tablespoons of the bacon fat, bacon, onion, apple cider vinegar, erythritol, garlic, and coffee to the insert. Stir to combine.

3. Cook uncovered for 3 to 4 hours on high, until the liquid has thickened and reduced.

4. Cool completely.

5. Store the bacon jam in the refrigerator in a sealed container for up to 3 weeks.

MAKE IT PALEO: The sweetener used in this condiment creates a jamlike profile, but you can use fruit instead of erythritol to produce a similar result. Add ½ cup raspberries to the slow cooker along with the rest of the ingredients.

ROASTED GARLIC

MAKES 2 CUPS / PREP TIME: 10 MINUTES / COOK TIME: 8 HOURS ON LOW

Roasted garlic is a culinary masterpiece. It is unbelievably fragrant, rich tasting, and silky smooth in texture. The scent of it roasting in your slow cooker might entice you to hang out in the kitchen until it is ready. Use it in place of garlic in other recipes to deepen the flavor of the dish.

6 HEADS GARLIC

¼ CUP EXTRA-VIRGIN OLIVE OIL

SALT, FOR SEASONING

1. Lay a large sheet of aluminum foil on your counter.
2. Cut the top off the heads of garlic, exposing the cloves. Place the garlic, cut side up, on the foil and drizzle them with the olive oil. Lightly season the garlic with salt.
3. Loosely fold the foil around the garlic to form a packet. Place the packet in the insert of the slow cooker.
4. Cover and cook on low for 8 hours.
5. Let the garlic cool for 10 minutes and then squeeze the cloves out of the papery skins.
6. Store the garlic in a sealed container in the refrigerator for up to 1 week.

PRECOOKING TIP: Blanch loose peeled garlic cloves for 5 minutes in simmering milk to reduce any bitterness, rinse them, and package them in the foil after drizzling them with olive oil and salt if you do not want to press the garlic out of the skins.

DAIRY-FREE
NUT-FREE
ALLERGEN-FREE
PALEO-FRIENDLY
QUICK PREP

KETO QUOTIENT

MACRONUTRIENTS
65% FAT
5% PROTEIN
30% CARBS

PER SERVING
(1 TABLESPOON)
CALORIES: 25
TOTAL FAT: 2G
PROTEIN: 0G
TOTAL CARBS: 2G
FIBER: 0G
NET CARBS: 2G
CHOLESTEROL: 0MG

SLOW-COOKER KETCHUP

MAKES 2 CUPS / PREP TIME: 10 MINUTES / COOK TIME: 6 TO 7 HOURS ON LOW

You might be wondering why you should go through the effort of making ketchup when you can just buy it at the grocery store. Prepared ketchup contains zero fat and protein and only 5 grams of total carbs, so this low-carb version is much better. The lovely tang in this bright condiment comes from the apple cider vinegar that is thought to be a weight-loss tool. Apple cider vinegar can help reduce blood-sugar spikes, and it increases the feeling of fullness. It can control cravings and overeating.

1 TABLESPOON EXTRA-VIRGIN OLIVE OIL

1 (28-OUNCE) CAN CRUSHED TOMATOES

½ CUP APPLE CIDER VINEGAR

¼ CUP GRANULATED ERYTHRITOL

1 SWEET ONION, FINELY CHOPPED

2 TEASPOONS MINCED GARLIC

¼ TEASPOON ALLSPICE

⅛ TEASPOON GROUND CLOVES

⅛ TEASPOON CELERY SALT

2 BAY LEAVES

1. Lightly grease the insert of the slow cooker with the olive oil.

2. Add the tomatoes, apple cider vinegar, erythritol, onion, garlic, allspice, cloves, celery salt, and bay leaves to the insert.

3. Cook uncovered for 6 to 7 hours on low, until thick.

4. Remove the bay leaves.

5. Use an immersion blender or a regular blender to purée the mixture.

6. Cool and transfer the ketchup to jars, seal, and refrigerate.

7. Store the ketchup in the refrigerator for up to 1 week or in the freezer for up to 2 months.

MAKE IT PALEO: Ketchup is often too sweet due to the added sugar and sweeteners, but you don't need to add the erythritol to produce a lovely condiment. Tomatoes have enough natural sugars in them, and the flavor is intensified when this ingredient is cooked for a long time in a slow cooker.

GOLDEN CARAMELIZED ONIONS

MAKES 3 CUPS / PREP TIME: 10 MINUTES / COOK TIME: 9 TO 10 HOURS ON LOW

The absolute best onions to caramelize are Vidalia, although some chefs might have a different opinion. Vidalia onions have a higher sugar content, which creates a lovely golden color faster when roasted and a richer taste than other onions. You can certainly use other onions such as Walla Walla or plain yellow if Vidalia onions are not available.

6 SWEET ONIONS, SLICED

¼ CUP EXTRA-VIRGIN OLIVE OIL

½ TEASPOON SALT

1. In a large bowl, toss together the onions, oil, and salt. Transfer the mixture to the insert of the slow cooker.

2. Cover and cook on low for 9 to 10 hours.

3. Serve, or store after cooling in a sealed container in the refrigerator for up to 5 days.

> **PRECOOKING TIP:** The onions will get sweet and thick when they are prepared in a slow cooker, but they will not become as caramelized as when first sautéed in a skillet. You can sauté the onions for about 15 minutes before placing them in the insert, tossing frequently, to create a richer finished condiment.

DAIRY-FREE
NUT-FREE
ALLERGEN-FREE
PALEO-FRIENDLY
QUICK PREP

KETO QUOTIENT

MACRONUTRIENTS
70% FAT
2% PROTEIN
28% CARBS

PER SERVING (¼ CUP)
CALORIES: 64
TOTAL FAT: 5G
PROTEIN: 1G
TOTAL CARBS: 5G
FIBER: 2G
NET CARBS: 3G
CHOLESTEROL: 0MG

GHEE

MAKES 2 CUPS / PREP TIME: 2 MINUTES / COOK TIME: 6 HOURS ON LOW

NUT-FREE
QUICK PREP

KETO QUOTIENT

MACRONUTRIENTS
100% FAT
0% PROTEIN
0% CARBS

PER SERVING
(1 TABLESPOON)
CALORIES: 100
TOTAL FAT: 11G
PROTEIN: 0G
TOTAL CARBS: 0G
FIBER: 0G
NET CARBS: 0G
CHOLESTEROL: 30MG

Clarified butter, the clear golden product served with your lobster or crab legs, and ghee are very similar. Clarified butter is unsalted butter that is heated until the milk solids and water separate, and then these elements are skimmed off, leaving just the fat. Ghee is unsalted butter that is heated for a long time over low heat until the milk solids and water are all cooked off. This means ghee is appropriate for those who are lactose intolerant.

1 POUND UNSALTED BUTTER, DICED

1. Place the butter in the insert of the slow cooker.
2. Cook on low with the lid set slightly open for 6 hours.
3. Pour the melted butter through a fine-mesh cheesecloth into a bowl.
4. Cool the ghee for 30 minutes and pour into a jar.
5. Store the ghee in the refrigerator for up to 2 weeks.

VARIATION TIP: Ghee can be flavored with different spices and herbs for interesting versions of the original product. Add sprigs of thyme or rosemary or a couple of teaspoons of coriander or cumin seed and simply strain out the additions when the ghee is done.

SPINACH-CHEESE SPREAD

MAKES 4 CUPS / PREP TIME: 10 MINUTES / COOK TIME: 5 TO 6 HOURS ON LOW

This recipe is very similar to the popular artichoke-and-spinach dip served in many restaurants and homes, so you will be familiar with the tempting flavor. You can whip up a batch and store it in the refrigerator for a quick snack or topping for eggs or poultry. You can also transfer the spread to a smaller crock, top it with a slice of cheese, and heat it up for a special-event snack.

1 TABLESPOON EXTRA-VIRGIN OLIVE OIL

8 OUNCES CREAM CHEESE

1 CUP SOUR CREAM

½ CUP SHREDDED CHEDDAR CHEESE

½ CUP SHREDDED MOZZARELLA CHEESE

½ CUP PARMESAN CHEESE

½ SWEET ONION, FINELY CHOPPED

2 TEASPOONS MINCED GARLIC

12 OUNCES CHOPPED SPINACH

1. Grease an 8-by-4-inch loaf pan with the olive oil.
2. In a large bowl, stir together the cream cheese, sour cream, Cheddar, mozzarella, Parmesan, onion, garlic, and spinach until well mixed.
3. Transfer the mixture to the loaf pan and place the pan in the insert of the slow cooker.
4. Cover and cook on low for 5 to 6 hours.
5. Serve warm.

> **VARIATION TIP:** Any dark leafy green, such as kale or Swiss chard, can be used in this tempting creamy creation. You can also add ½ cup chopped artichoke hearts for a traditional combination. This will add 2 grams of carbs to the finished dish.

NUT-FREE
QUICK PREP

KETO QUOTIENT

MACRONUTRIENTS
80% FAT
15% PROTEIN
5% CARBS

PER SERVING (½ CUP)
CALORIES: 245
TOTAL FAT: 21G
PROTEIN: 9G
TOTAL CARBS: 5G
FIBER: 1G
NET CARBS: 4G
CHOLESTEROL: 57MG

HOT CRAB SAUCE

MAKES 4 CUPS / PREP TIME: 10 MINUTES / COOK TIME: 5 TO 6 HOURS ON LOW

NUT-FREE
QUICK PREP

KETO QUOTIENT

MACRONUTRIENTS
70% FAT
20% PROTEIN
10% CARBS

PER SERVING (½ CUP)
CALORIES: 361
TOTAL FAT: 28G
PROTEIN: 17G
TOTAL CARBS: 10G
FIBER: 2G
NET CARBS: 8G
CHOLESTEROL: 88MG

Crab has a sweet, buttery taste that is luscious when paired with three kinds of cheeses and tangy sour cream in this recipe. Crabmeat is packed with vitamin B_{12}, so eating this sauce as a dip for a handful of vegetables as an afternoon snack ensures you have lots of energy for the evening. Add red pepper flakes to add a kick or lemon juice to brighten the flavor of the other ingredients.

8 OUNCES CREAM CHEESE

8 OUNCES GOAT CHEESE

1 CUP SOUR CREAM

½ CUP GRATED ASIAGO CHEESE

1 SWEET ONION, FINELY CHOPPED

1 TABLESPOON GRANULATED ERYTHRITOL

2 TEASPOONS MINCED GARLIC

12 OUNCES CRABMEAT, FLAKED

1 SCALLION, WHITE AND GREEN
PARTS, CHOPPED

1. In a large bowl, stir together the cream cheese, goat cheese, sour cream, Asiago cheese, onion, erythritol, garlic, crabmeat, and scallion until well mixed.

2. Transfer the mixture to an 8-by-4-inch loaf pan and place the pan in the insert of the slow cooker.

3. Cover and cook on low for 5 to 6 hours.

4. Serve warm.

ALLERGEN TIP: If you are allergic to shellfish, you can use chopped chicken instead with delicious results.

ENCHILADA SAUCE

MAKES 4 CUPS / PREP TIME: 10 MINUTES / COOK TIME: 7 TO 8 HOURS ON LOW

Unfortunately, you will not be eating enchiladas on the keto diet, but that shouldn't stop you from enjoying the sauce as an accompaniment for entrées and side dishes. The heat and intense tomato flavor pair well with chicken and beef, especially on a homemade burger served on a crisp lettuce leaf. Top the sauce with Cheddar cheese for a wonderful meal.

¼ CUP EXTRA-VIRGIN OLIVE OIL, DIVIDED

2 CUPS PURÉED TOMATOES

1 CUP WATER

1 SWEET ONION, CHOPPED

2 JALAPEÑO PEPPERS, CHOPPED

2 TEASPOONS MINCED GARLIC

2 TABLESPOONS CHILI POWDER

1 TEASPOON GROUND CORIANDER

1. Lightly grease the insert of the slow cooker with 1 tablespoon of the olive oil.

2. Place the remaining 3 tablespoons of the olive oil, tomatoes, water, onion, jalapeño peppers, garlic, chili powder, and coriander in the insert.

3. Cover and cook on low 7 to 8 hours.

4. Serve over poultry or meat. After cooling, store the sauce in a sealed container in the refrigerator for up to 1 week.

PRECOOKING TIP: For an utterly spectacular flavor, you can roast the tomatoes before adding them to the slow cooker. Just arrange about 10 halved tomatoes on a baking sheet, and place them in a 400°F oven for about 2 hours before puréeing them in a blender.

DAIRY-FREE
NUT-FREE
ALLERGEN-FREE
PALEO-FRIENDLY
QUICK PREP

KETO QUOTIENT

MACRONUTRIENTS
78% FAT
7% PROTEIN
15% CARBS

PER SERVING (½ CUP)
CALORIES: 92
TOTAL FAT: 8G
PROTEIN: 2G
TOTAL CARBS: 4G
FIBER: 2G
NET CARBS: 2G
CHOLESTEROL: 0MG

CREAMY ALFREDO SAUCE

MAKES 6 CUPS / PREP TIME: 5 MINUTES / COOK TIME: 6 HOURS ON LOW

NUT-FREE
QUICK PREP

KETO QUOTIENT

MACRONUTRIENTS
85% FAT
10% PROTEIN
5% CARBS

PER SERVING (½ CUP)
CALORIES: 280
TOTAL FAT: 27G
PROTEIN: 7G
TOTAL CARBS: 4G
FIBER: 0G
NET CARBS: 4G
CHOLESTEROL: 84MG

This is one of those simple recipes that will baffle chefs because a slow cooker really should not produce such a creamy and smooth sauce. Chefs spend hours perfecting the techniques required for Alfredo sauce, and you just get to set it and forget it. The gentle reduction creates a rich roasted garlic scent that will call your family to your dinner table as effectively as ringing a bell.

1 TABLESPOON EXTRA-VIRGIN OLIVE OIL

4 CUPS CHICKEN BROTH

2 CUPS HEAVY (WHIPPING) CREAM

3 TEASPOONS MINCED GARLIC

½ CUP BUTTER

1 CUP GRATED PARMESAN CHEESE

2 TABLESPOONS CHOPPED FRESH PARSLEY

FRESHLY GROUND BLACK PEPPER,
FOR SEASONING

1. Lightly grease the insert of the slow cooker with the olive oil.

2. Stir in the broth, heavy cream, and garlic until combined.

3. Cover and cook on low for 6 hours.

4. Whisk in the butter, Parmesan cheese, and parsley.

5. Season with pepper and serve.

VARIATION TIP: This sauce is meant to taste like a traditional Alfredo sauce, with lots of garlic and the sharp flavor of grated Parmesan. You can add different cheeses, such as goat cheese or Swiss, or other herbs to create a unique variation to use with vegetables and zucchini noodles or spooned over proteins.

QUESO SAUCE

MAKES 4 CUPS / PREP TIME: 10 MINUTES / COOK TIME: 3 TO 4 HOURS ON LOW

Queso is the Spanish word for "cheese," so it is an entirely appropriate name for this scrumptious and cheese-packed sauce. Try serving it as a dip for celery or cauliflower or as a topping for grilled chicken, beef, or pork. You can also spoon it over scrambled eggs for a flavor-packed breakfast.

1 TABLESPOON EXTRA-VIRGIN OLIVE OIL

12 OUNCES CREAM CHEESE

1 CUP SOUR CREAM

2 CUPS SALSA VERDE

1 CUP MONTEREY JACK CHEESE, SHREDDED

1. Lightly grease the insert of the slow cooker with the olive oil.
2. In a large bowl, stir together the cream cheese, sour cream, salsa verde, and Monterey Jack cheese, until blended.
3. Transfer the mixture to the insert.
4. Cover and cook on low for 3 to 4 hours.
5. Serve warm.

> **VARIATION TIP:** Salsa verde is a traditional creation made with tomatillos, jalapeño peppers, and lime. It is green, as the name suggests. You can use regular tomato-based salsa instead.

NUT-FREE
QUICK PREP

KETO QUOTIENT

MACRONUTRIENTS
81% FAT
13% PROTEIN
6% CARBS

PER SERVING (½ CUP)
CALORIES: 278
TOTAL FAT: 25G
PROTEIN: 9G
TOTAL CARBS: 4G
FIBER: 0G
NET CARBS: 4G
CHOLESTEROL: 72MG

CLASSIC BOLOGNESE SAUCE

SERVES 10 / PREP TIME: 15 MINUTES / COOK TIME: 7 TO 8 HOURS ON LOW

DAIRY-FREE
ALLERGEN-FREE
PALEO-FRIENDLY
QUICK PREP

KETO QUOTIENT

MACRONUTRIENTS
62% FAT
30% PROTEIN
8% CARBS

PER SERVING
CALORIES: 333
TOTAL FAT: 23G
PROTEIN: 25G
TOTAL CARBS: 9G
FIBER: 3G
NET CARBS: 6G
CHOLESTEROL: 98MG

It should be no surprise that Bolognese sauce originates from Bologna, Italy. This meaty creation is meant to simmer all day on the stove so that the beefy flavor is rich and the sauce thick. Slow cooking matures the sauce, creating an absolutely perfect marriage between the different meats, vegetables, and herbs.

3 TABLESPOONS EXTRA-VIRGIN
    OLIVE OIL, DIVIDED
1 POUND GROUND PORK
½ POUND GROUND BEEF
½ POUND BACON, CHOPPED
1 SWEET ONION, CHOPPED

1 TABLESPOON MINCED GARLIC
2 CELERY STALKS, CHOPPED
1 CARROT, CHOPPED
2 (28-OUNCE) CANS DICED TOMATOES
½ CUP COCONUT MILK
¼ CUP APPLE CIDER VINEGAR

1. Lightly grease the insert of the slow cooker with 1 tablespoon of the olive oil.

2. In a large skillet over medium-high heat, heat the remaining 2 tablespoons of the olive oil. Add the pork, beef, and bacon, and sauté until cooked through, about 7 minutes.

3. Stir in the onion and garlic and sauté for an additional 2 minutes.

4. Transfer the meat mixture to the insert and add the celery, carrot, tomatoes, coconut milk, and apple cider vinegar.

5. Cover and cook on low for 7 to 8 hours.

6. Serve, or cool completely, and store in the refrigerator in a sealed container for up to 4 days or in the freezer for 1 month.

VARIATION TIP: The mixture of pork and beef creates a slightly different taste from only using ground beef. Ground pork tends to be leaner than regular ground beef, so if you want to increase the fat grams in the sauce, use only 80 percent lean beef along with the bacon.

SIMPLE MARINARA SAUCE

SERVES 12 / PREP TIME: 10 MINUTES / COOK TIME: 7 TO 8 HOURS ON LOW

Marinara sauce is traditionally simmered very slowly on the back burner of the stove, wafting the enticing aroma of tomatoes, garlic, and herbs through the house. The slow cooker is the perfect tool to create this sauce with much less attention and time spent stirring. Marinara freezes beautifully for up to 2 months, so cool it in the refrigerator quickly, right in the insert, and transfer the sauce to sealable plastic freezer bags or containers.

3 TABLESPOONS EXTRA-VIRGIN OLIVE OIL, DIVIDED

2 (28-OUNCE) CANS CRUSHED TOMATOES

½ SWEET ONION, FINELY CHOPPED

2 TEASPOONS MINCED GARLIC

½ TEASPOON SALT

1 TABLESPOON CHOPPED FRESH BASIL

1 TABLESPOON CHOPPED FRESH OREGANO

1. Lightly grease the insert of the slow cooker with 1 tablespoon of the olive oil.

2. Add the remaining 2 tablespoons of the olive oil, tomatoes, onion, garlic, and salt to the insert, stirring to combine.

3. Cover and cook on low for 7 to 8 hours.

4. Remove the cover and stir in the basil and oregano.

5. Store the cooled sauce in a sealed container in the refrigerator for up to 1 week.

> **VARIATION TIP:** Tomato sauces are enhanced by whatever herbs and seasoning you add to the base ingredients. Red pepper flakes, thyme, parsley, and marjoram are all lovely additions if you want a different-tasting sauce.

DAIRY-FREE
NUT-FREE
ALLERGEN-FREE
PALEO-FRIENDLY
QUICK PREP

KETO QUOTIENT

MACRONUTRIENTS
54% FAT
7% PROTEIN
39% CARBS

PER SERVING (½ CUP)
CALORIES: 66
TOTAL FAT: 5G
PROTEIN: 1G
TOTAL CARBS: 7G
FIBER: 2G
NET CARBS: 5G
CHOLESTEROL: 0MG

CHICKEN BONE BROTH

MAKES 8 CUPS / PREP TIME: 15 MINUTES / COOK TIME: 24 HOURS ON LOW

DAIRY-FREE
NUT-FREE
ALLERGEN-FREE
PALEO-FRIENDLY
QUICK PREP

KETO QUOTIENT

MACRONUTRIENTS
55% FAT
24% PROTEIN
21% CARBS

PER SERVING (1 CUP)
CALORIES: 99
TOTAL FAT: 6G
PROTEIN: 6G
TOTAL CARBS: 5G
FIBER: 0G
NET CARBS: 5G
CHOLESTEROL: 7MG

Homemade chicken soup is a wonderful remedy for many ailments, including the common cold. Chicken bone broth contains a natural amino acid called cysteine that can improve breathing by thinning mucus in the lungs. So, whenever you have an extra chicken carcass, whip up a batch of this broth and keep it in the freezer for all of your recipes.

1 TABLESPOON EXTRA-VIRGIN OLIVE OIL
2 CHICKEN CARCASSES, SEPARATED INTO PIECES
2 GARLIC CLOVES, CRUSHED
1 CELERY STALK, CHOPPED
1 CARROT, CHOPPED

½ SWEET ONION, CUT INTO EIGHTHS
2 TABLESPOONS APPLE CIDER VINEGAR
2 BAY LEAVES
½ TEASPOON BLACK PEPPERCORNS
WATER

1. Lightly grease the insert of the slow cooker with the olive oil.

2. Place the chicken bones, garlic, celery, carrot, onion, apple cider vinegar, bay leaves, and peppercorns in the insert. Add water until the liquid reaches about 1½ inches from the top of the insert.

3. Cover and cook on low for about 24 hours.

4. Strain the broth through a fine-mesh cheesecloth and throw away the solids.

5. Store the broth in sealed containers in the refrigerator for up to 5 days or in the freezer for up to 1 month.

PRECOOKING TIP: As with any stock, roasting the bones before adding them produces a better end product. This is not a necessary step, but you will notice the difference in the taste of the broth.

HERBED VEGETABLE BROTH

MAKES 8 CUPS / PREP TIME: 15 MINUTES / COOK TIME: 8 HOURS ON LOW

Vegetable broth with a hint of herbs is the perfect liquid to use in fish recipes, side dishes, and vegetarian entrées. The black peppercorns add a bit of heat even if they are not crushed. White peppercorns can be used as well; they are black ones without their skin.

1 TABLESPOON EXTRA-VIRGIN OLIVE OIL

4 GARLIC CLOVES, CRUSHED

2 CELERY STALKS WITH GREENS, ROUGHLY CHOPPED

1 SWEET ONION, QUARTERED

1 CARROT, ROUGHLY CHOPPED

½ CUP CHOPPED PARSLEY

4 THYME SPRIGS

2 BAY LEAVES

½ TEASPOON BLACK PEPPERCORNS

½ TEASPOON SALT

8 CUPS WATER

1. Lightly grease the insert of the slow cooker with the olive oil.

2. Place the garlic, celery, onion, carrot, parsley, thyme, bay leaves, peppercorns, and salt in the insert. Add the water.

3. Cover and cook on low for about 8 hours.

4. Strain the broth through a fine-mesh cheesecloth and throw away the solids.

5. Store the broth in sealed containers in the refrigerator for up to 5 days or in the freezer for up to 1 month.

> **VARIATION TIP:** Any type of vegetable can be used to create a flavorful broth, so keep your peelings, ends, and herb sprigs to throw in whenever you want to make a batch. Broccoli and cauliflower stalks work very well after you have removed the florets for another recipe.

DAIRY-FREE
NUT-FREE
ALLERGEN-FREE
PALEO-FRIENDLY
QUICK PREP

KETO QUOTIENT

MACRONUTRIENTS
65% FAT
0% PROTEIN
35% CARBS

PER SERVING (1 CUP)
CALORIES: 27
TOTAL FAT: 2G
PROTEIN: 0G
TOTAL CARBS: 2G
FIBER: 0G
NET CARBS: 2G
CHOLESTEROL: 0MG

BEEF BONE BROTH

MAKES 8 CUPS / PREP TIME: 15 MINUTES / COOK TIME: 24 HOURS ON LOW

Beef bone broth is a staple ingredient for many people due to its nutritional benefits. Cooking this broth in a slow cooker is the best method. Do not omit the apple cider vinegar because it helps leach the minerals from the beef bones, providing nutrients. Bone broth can help support a strong immune system and fight inflammation in the body.

1 TABLESPOON EXTRA-VIRGIN OLIVE OIL

2 POUNDS BEEF BONES WITH MARROW

2 CELERY STALKS WITH GREENS, CHOPPED

1 CARROT, ROUGHLY CHOPPED

1 SWEET ONION, QUARTERED

4 GARLIC CLOVES, CRUSHED

2 TABLESPOONS APPLE CIDER VINEGAR

½ TEASPOON WHOLE BLACK PEPPERCORNS

½ TEASPOON SALT

2 BAY LEAVES

5 PARSLEY SPRIGS

4 THYME SPRIGS

WATER

1. Lightly grease the insert of the slow cooker with the olive oil.

2. Place the beef bones, celery, carrot, onion, garlic, apple cider vinegar, peppercorns, salt, bay leaves, parsley, and thyme in the insert. Add water until the liquid reaches about 1½ inches from the top.

3. Cover and cook on low for about 24 hours.

4. Strain the broth through a fine-mesh cheesecloth and throw away the solids.

5. Store the broth in sealed containers in the refrigerator for up to 5 days or in the freezer for up to 1 month.

PRECOOKING TIP: If you want to create a darker, richer broth, you can roast the bones in the oven for 30 minutes before placing them in the slow cooker. Preheat the oven to 350°F and add the celery, carrot, onion, and garlic to the roasting sheet as well.

CAROLINA BARBECUE SAUCE

MAKES 2 CUPS / PREP TIME: 10 MINUTES / COOK TIME: 3 HOURS ON LOW

Keto is a meat-heavy diet, so a delectable barbecue sauce to dip into or brush on is a valuable addition to your kitchen. The spicing found in this version creates a bit of heat. You can increase this fiery finish with cayenne or a pinch of red pepper flakes. A tablespoon of liquid smoke is also a lovely addition.

3 TABLESPOONS EXTRA-VIRGIN OLIVE OIL, DIVIDED

2 (6-OUNCE) CANS TOMATO PASTE

½ CUP APPLE CIDER VINEGAR

½ CUP WATER

¼ CUP GRANULATED ERYTHRITOL

1 TABLESPOON SMOKED PAPRIKA

1 TEASPOON GARLIC POWDER

1 TEASPOON ONION POWDER

½ TEASPOON CHILI POWDER

¼ TEASPOON SALT

1. Grease the insert of the slow cooker with 1 tablespoon olive oil.

2. In a large bowl, whisk together the tomato paste, remaining olive oil, vinegar, water, erythritol, paprika, garlic powder, onion powder, chili powder, and salt until blended.

3. Pour the mixture into a slow cooker insert.

4. Cover and cook on low for 3 hours.

5. After cooling, store the sauce in a container in the refrigerator for up to 2 weeks.

> **MAKE IT PALEO:** Omit the erythritol from the sauce and add ½ cup puréed peach. The sauce will be less sweet overall, but will still have a hint of sweetness to offset the smoky heat of the other ingredients.

DAIRY-FREE
NUT-FREE
ALLERGEN-FREE
QUICK PREP

KETO QUOTIENT

MACRONUTRIENTS
58% FAT
6% PROTEIN
36% CARBS

PER SERVING
(1 TABLESPOON)
CALORIES: 21
TOTAL FAT: 1G
PROTEIN: 0G
TOTAL CARBS: 2G
FIBER: 1G
NET CARBS: 1G
CHOLESTEROL: 0MG

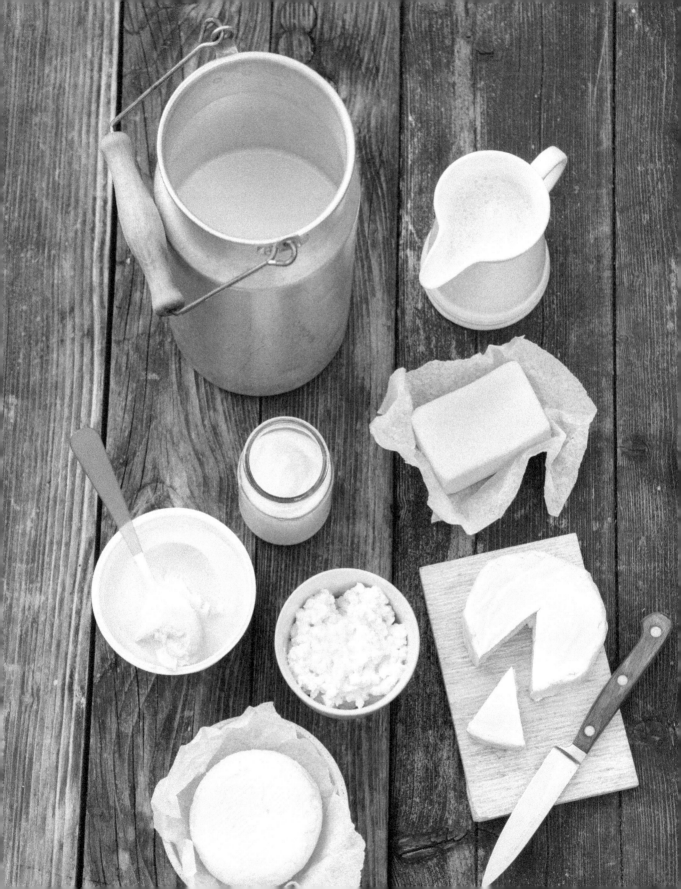

THE DIRTY DOZEN AND THE CLEAN FIFTEEN

A nonprofit and environmental watchdog organization called the Environmental Working Group (EWG) looks at data supplied by the US Department of Agriculture (USDA) and the Food and Drug Administration (FDA) about pesticide residues. Each year, it compiles a list of the lowest and highest pesticide loads found in commercial crops. You can use these lists to decide which fruits and vegetables to buy organic to minimize your exposure to pesticides and which conventional produce is considered safe enough to eat. This does not mean they are pesticide-free, though, so wash these (and all) fruits and vegetables thoroughly.

These lists change every year, so make sure you look up the most recent one before you fill your shopping cart. You'll find the most recent lists as well as a guide to pesticides in produce at EWG.org/FoodNews.

THE DIRTY DOZEN

Apples • Celery • Cherry tomatoes • Cucumbers • Grapes
Nectarines (imported) • Peaches • Potatoes • Snap peas (imported)
Spinach • Strawberries • Sweet bell peppers
(Kale/Collard greens • Hot peppers)**

** In addition to the dirty dozen, the EWG added two produce items contaminated with highly toxic organophosphate insecticides.

THE CLEAN FIFTEEN

Asparagus • Avocados • Cabbage • Cantaloupes (domestic) • Cauliflower
Eggplant • Grapefruit • Kiwifruit • Mangos • Onions • Papayas • Pineapples
Sweet corn • Sweet peas (frozen) • Sweet potatoes

CONVERSION TABLES

VOLUME EQUIVALENTS (LIQUID)

US STANDARD	US STANDARD (OUNCES)	METRIC (APPROXIMATE)
2 tablespoons	1 fl. oz.	30 mL
¼ cup	2 fl. oz.	60 mL
½ cup	4 fl. oz.	120 mL
1 cup	8 fl. oz.	240 mL
1½ cups	12 fl. oz.	355 mL
2 cups or 1 pint	16 fl. oz.	475 mL
4 cups or 1 quart	32 fl. oz.	1 L
1 gallon	128 fl. oz.	4 L

OVEN TEMPERATURES

FAHRENHEIT (F)	CELSIUS (C) (APPROXIMATE)
250°F	120°C
300°F	150°C
325°F	165°C
350°F	180°C
375°F	190°C
400°F	200°C
425°F	220°C
450°F	230°C

VOLUME EQUIVALENTS (DRY)

US STANDARD	METRIC (APPROXIMATE)
⅛ teaspoon	0.5 mL
¼ teaspoon	1 mL
½ teaspoon	2 mL
¾ teaspoon	4 mL
1 teaspoon	5 mL
1 tablespoon	15 mL
¼ cup	59 mL
⅓ cup	79 mL
½ cup	118 mL
⅔ cup	156 mL
¾ cup	177 mL
1 cup	235 mL
2 cups or 1 pint	475 mL
3 cups	700 mL
4 cups or 1 quart	1 L
½ gallon	2 L
1 gallon	4 L

WEIGHT EQUIVALENTS

US STANDARD	METRIC (APPROXIMATE)
½ ounce	15 g
1 ounce	30 g
2 ounces	60 g
4 ounces	115 g
8 ounces	225 g
12 ounces	340 g
16 ounces or 1 pound	455 g

RECITE INDEX

INDEX

CPSIA information can be obtained
at www.ICGtesting.com
Printed in the USA
BVHW02s1623301117
501628BV00001B/1/P